Designing Telehealth for an Aging Population

A Human Factors Perspective

Human Factors & Aging Series

Series Editors
Wendy A. Rogers and Arthur D. Fisk
School of Psychology
Georgia Institute of Technology – Atlanta, Georgia

Published Titles

Designing Displays for Older Adults
Richard Pak and Anne McLaughlin

Designing for Older Adults: Principles and Creative Human Factors Approaches, Second Edition
Arthur D. Fisk, Wendy A. Rogers, Neil Charness, Sara J. Czaja, and Joseph Sharit

Designing Telehealth for an Aging Population: A Human Factors Perspective
Neil Charness, George Demiris, and Elizabeth Krupinski

Forthcoming Titles

Aging and Skill Acquisition: Designing Training Programs for Older Adults
Sara J. Czaja and Joseph Sharit

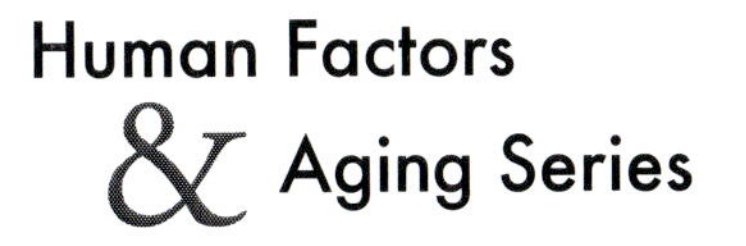

Designing Telehealth for an Aging Population

A Human Factors Perspective

Neil Charness
George Demiris
Elizabeth Krupinski

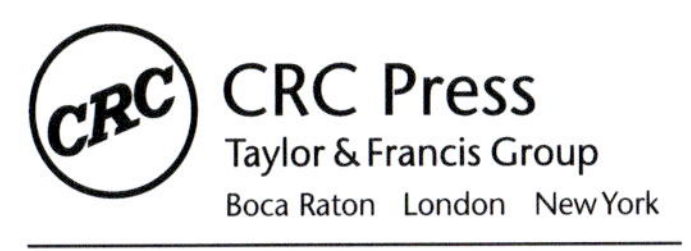

CRC Press is an imprint of the
Taylor & Francis Group, an **informa** business

CRC Press
Taylor & Francis Group
6000 Broken Sound Parkway NW, Suite 300
Boca Raton, FL 33487-2742

Printed in the United States of America on acid-free paper
Version Date: 20110822

International Standard Book Number: 978-1-4398-2529-7 (Paperback)

Visit the Taylor & Francis Web site at
http://www.taylorandfrancis.com

and the CRC Press Web site at
http://www.crcpress.com

Contents

Preface

Telehealth pertains to the exchange of health information and delivery of health services using electronic communications to improve the health and well-being of people across the spectrum of ages, locations, and health conditions. The practice of telehealth often involves new ways for patients and health care providers to interact and communicate to achieve the same or better outcomes than with traditional face-to-face health care. Our goal for this book, therefore, is to provide a brief primer on the human factors issues that can influence how older adults interact with telehealth systems. We also strive to follow the philosophy in this series of eschewing traditional academic writing (that cites research articles for each assertion). Instead we try to provide a distillation of our experience in this area in the form of basic observations and principles. We do provide suggested readings for those seeking to track down the research behind our recommendations.

We take inspiration from our association with the Human Factors Special Interest Group in the American Telemedicine Association, an association which has been at the forefront of promoting telemedicine in the United States and internationally. Our belief is that by paying attention to human factors principles, this new discipline can be much more successful in fitting telehealth systems to the needs of older users, whether in their role as health care providers or as consumers of health care.

Neil Charness
Elizabeth Krupinski
George Demiris

Acknowledgments

This work was supported in part by a grant to Neil Charness from the National Institutes of Health/National Institute on Aging (3 P01 AG 17211) under the auspices of the Center for Research and Education on Aging and Technology Enhancement (CREATE; www.create-center.org); a grant to Elizabeth Krupinski from Health Resources & Services Administration (HRSA)/Office for the Advancement of Telehealth (OAT) (G22IT16262); and a grant to George Demiris from the National Institutes of Health/National Institute of Nursing Research (R21NR01074).

Authors

Neil Charness is William G. Chase professor of psychology and an associate of the Pepper Institute on Aging and Public Policy at Florida State University, Tallahassee. He received his BA from McGill University, Montreal, Quebec, and MS and PhD from Carnegie Mellon University, Pittsburgh, Pennsylvania. Prior to coming to Florida, he was on the faculty at Wilfrid Laurier University, Waterloo, and the University of Waterloo in Canada. Neil's research focuses on human factors approaches to aging and technology use, older driver and pedestrian safety, and age and expert performance. Neil is a Fellow of the Association of Psychological Science, American Psychological Association (APA), Canadian Psychological Association (CPA), and the Gerontological Society of America, and is an honorary member of the International Society for Gerontechnology. He is a past editor of the psychology section of the *Canadian Journal on Aging/Revue Canadienne du Vieillissement*, and a past president of Adult Development and Aging Divisions of APA and CPA. He is currently chair of the Human Factors Special Interest Group of the American Telemedicine Association.

Elizabeth Krupinski is a professor at the University of Arizona in the departments of radiology, psychology, and public health, and she is vice chair of research in radiology. She received her undergraduate degree from Cornell University, MA from Montclair State College, and PhD from Temple University, all in experimental psychology. Her main interests are in medical image perception, assessment of observer performance, medical decision-making, and human factors. She is associate director of evaluation for the Arizona Telemedicine Program. She has published extensively in these areas and has presented at conferences nationally and internationally. She serves on the editorial boards of a number of journals in both radiology and telemedicine, and on review panels for the National Institutes of Health (NIH), Department of Defense (DoD), Food and Drug Administration (FDA), and the Telemedicine & Techhnology Research Center (TATRC). She is past chair of the Society for Photographic Instrumentation Engineers (SPIE) Medical Imaging Conference, past president of the American Telemedicine Association, and chair of the Society for Imaging Informatics in Medicine.

George Demiris is an associate professor of biobehavioral nursing and health systems at the School of Nursing and Biomedical and Health Informatics at the School of Medicine, University of Washington, Seattle. He is the graduate program director of Biomedical and Health Informatics at the School of Medicine and the director of the clinical informatics and patient centered technologies at the School of Nursing. He obtained his MSc in medical informatics from the University of Heidelberg, Germany, and his PhD in health informatics from the University of Minnesota. His research interests include the design and evaluation of home-based technologies for older adults and patients with chronic conditions and disabilities, smart homes and ambient assisted living applications, and the use of telehealth in home care and hospice. He is the chair of the International Medical Informatics Association (IMIA) Working Group on Smart Homes and Ambient Assisted Living, the past chair of the Human Factors Special Interest Group of the American Telemedicine Association (ATA), and the lead convener of the Technology and Aging Special Interest Group of the Gerontological Society of America (GSA).

chapter 1

Introduction and Purpose of This Volume

1.1 Definitions of Telemedicine and Telehealth

There are a large number of terms used somewhat interchangeably in the nascent field of remote health care. Popular ones, in order of frequency of occurrence (e.g., using Google's Ngram book search or by searching for words on the Internet), include telemedicine, telehealth, and e-health. A short definition for the field would be: the remote provision of health care services and education by means of information and communications technology. The term telemedicine more narrowly applies to health care and education provided by professionals in the field of medicine. The rise of the Internet has changed the health care dissemination process enormously and has led to the creation of terms such as telehealth and e-health. Some authors distinguish the two primary terms of telemedicine and telehealth as follows:

> If telehealth is understood to mean the integration of telecommunications systems into the practice of protecting and promoting health while telemedicine is the incorporation of these systems into curative medicine, then it must be acknowledged that telehealth corresponds more closely to the international activities of WHO in the field of public health. It covers education for health, public and community health, health systems development and epidemiology, whereas telemedicine is orientated more towards the clinical aspect. (Darkins & Cary, 2000, p. 2–3)

The journal *Telemedicine and e-Health* uses the following definition (Bashur et al., 2009): "Telemedicine technology embodies the electronic acquisition, processing, dissemination, storage, retrieval, and exchange of information for the purpose of promoting health, preventing disease, treating the sick, managing chronic illness, rehabilitating the disabled, and protecting public health and safety." (*Telemedicine and e-Health* 15(6): July/August 2009. doi: 10.1089/tmj.2009.9960, p. 2)

In summary, traditional health care has been delivered through in-person, real-time interactions between one or more care providers and a care recipient. Telehealth systems enable the provision of many aspects of health care either partially or completely by remote providers using both real-time and store-and-forward technologies. In this volume we will use terms such as telemedicine, telehealth, and e-health somewhat interchangeably.

The last century has seen enormous progress in one important measure of health: life expectancy. As an example, in the United States, life expectancy at birth has increased from about 47 years in 1900 to about 78 years in 2010. Falling death rates coupled with falling birth rates from the mid-1960s onward have resulted in an aging population. Aging is now a worldwide phenomenon, as many countries shift from high birth rates and high death rates to lower birth rates and much lower death rates. Japan is now the oldest country in the world, in terms of the percentage of its population over the age of 65, and has a life expectancy at birth of almost 83 years. Although progress on a critical index such as life expectancy is to be welcomed, an aging population presents numerous challenges to society. Perhaps the most important is that increased longevity is associated with an increased incidence of chronic diseases. The Centers for Disease Control and Prevention's definition of chronic diseases is that they are "noncommunicable illnesses that are prolonged in duration, do not resolve spontaneously, and are rarely cured completely," (accessed July 15, 2009, http://www.cdc.gov/nccdphp/publications/AAG/chronic.htm). Examples would be diseases such as hypertension, mental disorders, respiratory disease, arthritis, diabetes, and heart disease. People with chronic disorders accounted for nearly 90% of the total health care expenditures in the United States in 2005 (Machlin, Cohen, & Beauregard, 2008).

Another remarkable change seen in the United States has been the shift away from providing medical care through hospitals and doctor's offices in part because of the very high cost of providing services in those settings. As a result of such cost-shifting, patients are increasingly being called on to manage their own care, particularly for chronic conditions, in their homes or other community settings.

Over the last two centuries there has also been striking progress in the development of, and particularly in the dissemination of, information and communication technologies (ICT), starting with the widespread adoption of the telephone in the early 20th century and the mobile phone in the 21st century. Even more impressive have been the advances in health care technology; for instance, in our ability to peer into the human body noninvasively (x-ray, ultrasound, PET, EEG, MEG, and fMRI technology) to monitor both structural and functional aspects of health status. It is now possible to monitor many critical physiological and psychological functions remotely, including from homes. It is also possible to use the vastly improved communication infrastructure in place to transmit such information around the planet and even beyond to support humans in space. In fact, many advanced technologies for remote physiological monitoring were initially developed to support human space flight missions.

There is now an unprecedented opportunity to employ new technology developed in the health care field to provide more convenient and, hopefully, more efficient health care services to people in their homes. As well, there are opportunities to improve the delivery of health care to settings such as remote, isolated communities, and even to hostile environments such as disaster sites and battlefields. Finally, health care is a rapidly changing field. Best practice guidelines for everything from diagnosis to treatment are changing as advances are made in health care knowledge. Consequently, health care practitioners need continuing education. Modern telecommunication networks and particularly the Internet can provide efficient access to such knowledge for practitioners located in remote areas.

To ensure the success of these technological advances, designers and developers must attend to the human factors involved in their use. The goal for this volume is to provide a primer on how human factors and ergonomics tools can contribute to the success of telehealth. Hence, the book provides relevant information about human capabilities, guidelines for telehealth design, and tutorials on human factors methodologies that can aid in the successful development, deployment, and maintenance of telehealth technology.

1.2 *Human Factors and Ergonomics: Definitions*

There are some common themes in the various definitions of human factors and ergonomics. Both the International Ergonomics Association and the Human Factors and Ergonomics Society define ergonomics (or human factors) as "the scientific discipline concerned with the understanding of interactions among humans and other elements of a system, and the profession that applies theory, principles, data, and other methods to design in order to optimize human well-being and overall system performance" (see Human Factors and Ergonomics Society, What is human factors/ergonomics? http://www.hfes.org/Web/AboutHFES/about.html, and the International Ergonomics Association, What is ergonomics? http://www.iea.cc/01_what/What%20is%20Ergonomics.html). The influential *Handbook of Human Factors and Ergonomics* (Salvendy, 2006) indicated that the focus for this discipline is on "the nature of human-artifact interactions, viewed from the unified perspective of the science, engineering, design, technology, and management of human-compatible systems, including a variety of natural and artificial products, processes, and living environments" (p. 4).

In brief, this discipline is concerned with improving the fit between humans and the tools/technologies that they employ and the environments that they inhabit. A basic assumption is that human capabilities set limits on how successfully people can interact with the world in general, and with human-designed tools and environments in particular. If those limits are exceeded by system demands, interactions may become unsafe, unproductive, or unpleasant.

A particularly important finding is that humans are diverse in terms of features such as size, weight, shape, and for perceptual and cognitive abilities, but many of their capabilities will vary predictably with factors such as age (e.g., size, perceptual and cognitive capabilities) and gender (e.g., body dimensions). Because designers can often predict who the users of a product or service will be, it is possible to make use of knowledge of population characteristics to design within reasonable limits for those users. However, when it comes to health care, particularly in the case of acute disorders (e.g., injuries, diseases such as influenza) the entire population is at risk. In this volume we restrict consideration to aging adults, recognizing that they are a very diverse population by themselves. Although there is no magical age when someone becomes old, the convention we will follow is to use age 65 as a marker for considering someone to be an older adult. "Old" is a moving target. For example, the U.S. Census Bureau population pyramids for the year 1900 end at age 75+, though categories extend to age 95+ for projections to 2050. Older adults are disproportionately afflicted with chronic conditions such as diabetes, cancer, heart disease, and Alzheimer's disease, and hence are likely candidates for telehealth services.

1.3 *Person–Environment Fit: Why a Human Factors Approach Is Helpful*

A useful framework for understanding person–environment fit is shown in Figure 1.1. This framework highlights a few important principles. Users vary in their capabilities, often in predictable ways (age, education, and technical experience being mediators of capabilities). The primary ones we consider are the abilities to perceive information from the environment, to interpret and plan based on it, and then to carry out actions to achieve some task goal. The tool or environment poses challenges to the user's capabilities. If the demands and capabilities are in balance, then the user can efficiently, safely, and comfortably achieve his or her goal. When the demands exceed user capabilities, then task performance will suffer. Good design ensures that system demands fit with user capabilities.

Consider a telehealth tool such as a desktop-based videoconferencing unit. It usually has hardware and software components, such as a screen to

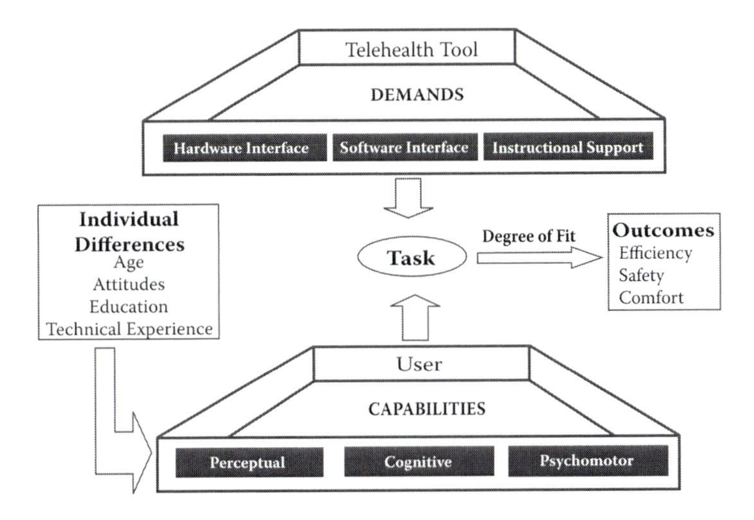

Figure 1.1 Capability-Demand Framework. (Reprinted with permission from *The Role of Human Factors in Home Health Care: Workshop Summary* by the National Academy of Sciences, 2010, courtesy of the National Academies Press, Washington, DC, from http://books.nap.edu/openbook.php?record_id=12927&page=78.)

convey visual images and text, sound emitting (headphones or speakers) and recording (microphone) components to convey auditory information, physical buttons to press, etc. As well, there is a software interface that organizes the type and sequence of information being received from and transmitted to the user. There are usually also materials providing instructional support, such as a manual (paper or electronic) or help system. This system makes demands on user capabilities, such as on their vision (size of text, image), hearing (intensity and clarity of sound relative to background noise), cognition (recalling how to carry out sequences of activities), and psychomotor ability (degree of fine motor control needed to adjust aspects of the system). The extent to which system demands can be met by user capabilities is termed the degree of fit. Degree of fit, in turn, determines the success of the interaction (assuming that the product is not defective to begin with). If demands are too great, the person may fail to complete the task successfully or complete it in a very inefficient fashion. Use of a system provides experience of varying levels of satisfaction with the interaction that can affect willingness to use the system in the future.

Users vary in terms of the knowledge and skills that they bring to bear in learning to use the system effectively. Factors such as their age, attitudes toward technology, and education level play an important role in the ability to interact with a system. People differ in their perceptual capabilities. For instance, older adults suffer from presbyopia (farsightedness), making focus on fine visual features difficult without corrective lenses.

They also are likely to suffer from some loss in sensitivity to sounds, particularly those components at higher frequencies (pitch). People differ in their cognitive capabilities. They may suffer from declines in working memory capacity that make it difficult to remember long sequences of actions required to operate the system. People differ in their psychomotor capabilities. Tremor in the hands may complicate physical interaction with a system. This analysis of human–technology interaction is a good start, but also incomplete.

If one considers that a system such as that shown above will involve interacting with a distant care provider, such as a physician or nurse, then other human–human interaction factors come into play such as expectations on the part of the user about the nature of the health care interaction. Cultural and educational differences as well as unique personal history factors may set expectations that play into how satisfying the interaction is with the distant health care provider. A similar set of issues arise for the health care provider in terms of interacting with the client. Thus, to design the whole system to work well, it is necessary to understand not just the technical components but also the human components.

1.4 Error

"To err is human, to forgive is divine." As the quote from Alexander Pope indicates, humans make mistakes (mental as well as physical ones). Such mistakes can sometimes be deadly in the health care field, as the Institute of Medicine report indicated, citing hospital-related errors as producing 90,000+ preventable fatalities yearly in the United States (Kohn, Korrigan, & Donaldson, 2000). Systems should be designed to be forgiving of errors, rather than hoping for divine intervention to avoid them. To quote the Roman philosopher Seneca, "Errare humanum est perseverare diabolicum." ("To err is human, to persist is the devil.") Well-designed systems should assume that people will make mistakes but permit them to recover from incorrect actions before they encounter a catastrophic outcome. Usability testing is a powerful human factors methodology for uncovering flaws in design that could lead to unsatisfactory (or even deadly) interactions.

1.5 Demographics of Health Care Utilization by an Aging Population

Health status is negatively correlated with age. One example can be seen in Figure 1.2 showing trends across age groups at 7-year intervals since 1995 for the U.S. population rating their general health status. Points represent the percent of each age group that rates their health as fair or poor

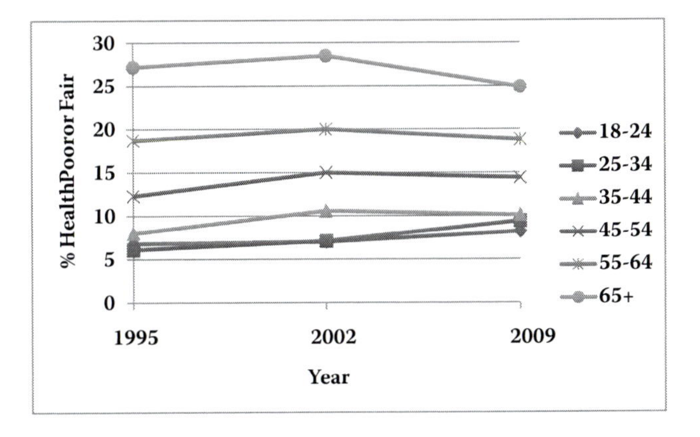

Figure 1.2 Age and time trends for general health status rated as fair or poor in the United States. (Data from the Behavioral Risk Factor Surveillance System (BRFSS), Centers for Disease Control and Prevention (CDC). *Behavioral Risk Factor Surveillance System Survey Questionnaire,* Atlanta, Georgia: U.S. Department of Health and Human Services, Centers for Disease Control and Prevention, 1995, 2002, 2009. Accessed March 8, 2011, http://apps.nccd.cdc.gov/brfss/age.asp?yr=1995&state=US&qkey=1100&grp=0.)

using a health rating scale with the labels excellent, very good, good, fair, and poor.

In general, the age group trends across years are for better health ratings (smaller percentages in the fair and poor categories) except for the two youngest age cohorts. Nonetheless, there is a marked increase in ratings of poorer health status as age increases beyond age 45 at every time point. Nearly a quarter of those age 65+ report being in fair or poor health status compared to less than 10% for those below the age of 45.

One reason for focusing on aging in this volume is that increased age is associated with an increased probability of incurring the types of chronic health conditions that may be well-managed remotely using telehealth technologies. A typical function can be seen in Figure 1.3.

Although chronic conditions account for much of the expenditure burden for health care (about 90% of expenditures in the United States are on behalf of those with chronic conditions), it is useful to note that illness arises at all ages, particularly for acute episodes such as contracting influenza. Even for such acute disorders it may be preferable for the afflicted person to engage with a health professional while at home via videoconferencing equipment supplemented by remote vital sign monitoring equipment rather than, for example, being forced to travel to an office and running the risk of being infected or infecting others while in the office. What type of infrastructure would it take to support those remote interactions? These issues are addressed in Chapters 2 and 3.

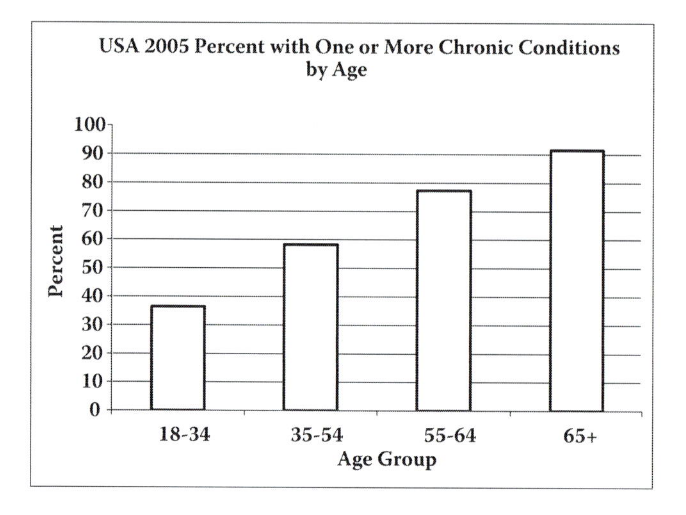

Figure 1.3 Prevalence of one or more chronic health conditions by age group. (Based on data from Machlin, Cohen and Beauregard, 2005.)

1.6 Population Aging and Health Care Profession Aging

A good indication of the aging of the population worldwide is provided by past and projected numbers of older adults, age 65+ and age 85+, in the Organisation for Economic Co-operation and Development (OECD) countries (34 economically advanced nations such as Japan, Italy, Canada, United States, Czech Republic, Australia, Turkey; http://www.oecd.org/pages/0,3417,en_36734052_36761800_1_1_1_1_1,00.html). Figure 1.4 shows the trends, namely more than a tripling from 1980 to 2050 for those ages 65-plus, and a doubling for those 85-plus.

Such projections, coupled with the chronic condition prevalence by age shown in Figure 1.3, imply that there will be a great need for cost effective health care provision in many countries. Telehealth technologies could play an important role in coping with rising demand for health care combined with an anticipated shrinking health care workforce in the years to come. Such technologies will fulfill their promise only when they can be tailored to fit the needs of both the user and the provider communities.

Health care providers are aging along with the general population and more so for certain professions. For instance, a 2008 survey of U.S. nurses found that the median age was about 46 years (U.S. Department of Health and Human Services, 2008, accessed March 9, 2011, http://bhpr.hrsa.gov/healthworkforce/rnsurvey/2008/), and nearly one in three physicians in the United States was age 55 or older in 2005 (Association of

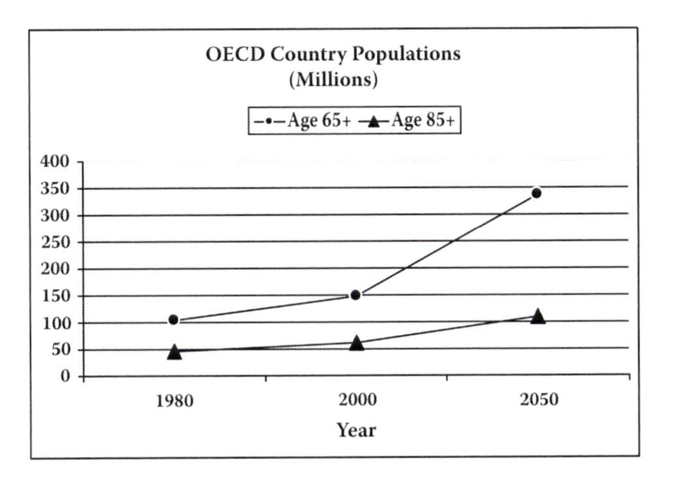

Figure 1.4 Projections for older adult populations in OECD countries. Source: OECD Demographic and Labour Force database, used in OECD, 2007, Society at a Glance: OECD Social Indicators 2006, accessed Oct. 23, 2009, http://www.oecd.org/dataoecd/52/31/38123085.xls.)

American Medical Colleges, 2006). The median age of the U.S. labor force was about 40 years of age in 2007 (Toosi, 2007). Physician age is also high in other countries. Canadian physicians had an average age of 49.7 years in 2009 (accessed March 9, 2011, http://www.cihi.ca/CIHI-ext-portal/internet/en/Document/spending+and+health+workforce/workforce/physicians/RELEASE_02DEC10) and German physicians averaged 51.3 years in 2003 (accessed March 9, 2011, http://www.biomedcentral.com/content/pdf/1471-2296-7-47.pdf). Hence telehealth systems also need to be designed to support older health care workers.

1.7 *Plan for the Book*

This chapter provides an overview of some of the critical issues concerning telehealth with an aging population. Next we describe the characteristics of an aging health care user (Chapter 2), focusing on capabilities in perception, cognition, and psychomotor performance. We follow this with Chapter 3, characterizing the health care environment in which telehealth equipment is typically deployed. Then we briefly discuss human factors issues for the main branches of telemedicine (Chapter 4). We present guidelines in Chapter 5. In Chapters 6 and 7 we provide some tutorials on a variety of topics (usability testing, setting up diagnostics, issues in health status monitoring, focus group methodology) that can be useful to practitioners. We end with a look into the future for this field in Chapter 8.

1.8 Suggested Readings

Darkins, A.W., & Cary, M.A. (2000). *Telemedicine and Telehealth: Principles, Policies, Performance and Pitfalls*. New York: Springer.

Kohn, L.T., Corrigan, J.M., & Donaldson, M.S. (2000). *To Err is Human: Building a Safer Health System*. Washington, DC: National Academy Press (http://www.nap.edu/catalog/9728.html).

Salvendy, G. (2006). *Handbook of Human Factors and Ergonomics*, 3rd ed. Hoboken, NJ: Wiley.

Stronge, A.J., Rogers, W.A., & Fisk, A.D. (2007). Human factors considerations in implementing telemedicine systems to accommodate older adults. *Journal of Telemedicine and Telecare*, 13, 1–3.

chapter 2

Know the Health Care User

The so-called first commandment of human factors is said to be "know thy user." That is, one must understand the capabilities and motivations of the user in order to design appropriately. Health care users, particularly older users, come in many shapes, sizes, colors, and most importantly, capabilities. The chapter begins with an overview of capabilities that can significantly influence interactions with telehealth technology. It ends with recommendations for design.

2.1 Perception

The first point of contact for interaction with a health care device or system is through the perceptual system. Perceptual systems encompass vision, hearing and balance, touch/haptics, temperature, smell, and taste. The latter two will not be reviewed because they are not typically used to convey telehealth information. However, although the latter might not seem to be particularly relevant to health care, taste and smell can seriously impact willingness to adhere to a procedure. For instance, preparation for a colonoscopy procedure involves consumption of large volumes of salty fluids. Smells and tastes can evoke negative emotions (such as conditioned aversions from earlier procedures) that can impact the success of the current procedure. The general findings on smell and taste are that these senses diminish in sensitivity as people age.

2.1.1 Vision

On surveys asking about concerns about aging, older adults identify loss of vision as one of their greatest fears (though dementia is usually an even bigger concern). Vision is the most important long-range perceptual system, providing information about distant objects in the environment. Some activities are currently impossible to carry out without vision, such as driving a motor vehicle (though this will change with further development of autonomous vehicles). Many technology artifacts require vision to encode and respond to information on screen displays (e.g., a digital thermometer or a blood pressure device). A good design principle is to allow for redundant output of information; for instance, provide both visual and auditory output.

Visual acuity, the ability to perceive fine detail, changes systematically in adulthood as a function of normative changes in the eye–brain system. The earliest noticeable change, usually in the decade of the 40s, is loss of focusing power in the lens. Focal power is lost due in part to changes in the musculature that controls the curvature of the lens (flattening out or bulging of the lens) coupled with changes in the size of the lens, which continues to add crystalline layers, thereby thickening across the lifespan and making the structure less flexible. The end result is that accommodative power to focus on near objects is lost. The inability to focus on near objects is termed presbyopia. The closest near point for focus tends to move out away from the viewer. People become more farsighted with increasing age. This change is best illustrated by "arm's length" reading distance for print before the middle-aged adult finally accedes to wearing corrective lenses (e.g., bifocals, progressive lenses, specialized contact lenses) to enable comfortable reading at nearer distances.

However, many situations, such as reading print from computer screens or numbers on a thermometer, may make visual demands that are not well-met by normal corrective lenses and hence can lead to eye strain and performance decline. Not all individuals adjust well to progressive lenses that provide a gradient where, if the eye is properly directed, nearly all points in the visual field can be brought into sharp focus. Thus the size of visual detail, such as print or icons, can be an important limiting factor in whether someone can read a display. As an example, mobile phone technology is increasingly being used to convey health information. Small mobile phone displays may be difficult to read for those with presbyopia. Although the trend in smartphones is toward the use of screens that are larger, with higher contrast and higher resolution, there is an open question about how usable they will be for older adults, particularly those with visual impairments.

One would think that if visual details are too small for older eyes, the person can always just move the object closer to the eye (e.g., that thermometer reading). However, remember that as objects move closer to the eye than the presbyopic focus point (or the corrected focus point with a bifocal lens), they will become blurry and illegible. Simply expecting older adults to put the object closer to their eyes to see fine visual detail better may not solve the problem (unless they are nearsighted, myopic, to begin with and take off their reading glasses). Magnifying lenses can help, but they may not always be easily accessible. Fortunately, many screen-based devices can alter the size of the objects in the display, though many people will not necessarily know how to do this. (How many readers have changed the default font size on their smartphones?)

Increased age is also associated with more serious visual diseases such as the formation of cataracts (opacities on the lens), abnormal buildup of pressure in the eye that can damage the retina (glaucoma), and

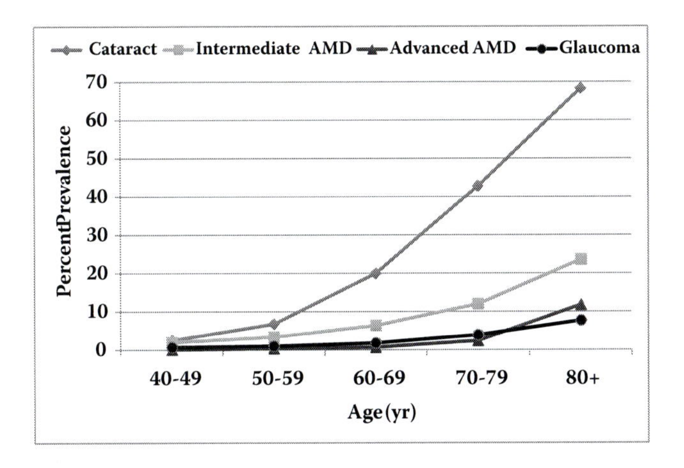

Figure 2.1 United States prevalence of visual disorders by age. (Data from the National Eye Institute, accessed Feb. 3, 2011, http://www.nei.nih.gov/eyedata/pbd_tables.asp.)

age-related macular degeneration (AMD; degeneration in the part of the retina responsible for high acuity daylight vision). The prevalence of these disorders in the United States can be seen in Figure 2.1.

Cataracts can be remedied with surgery (lens replacement) and some forms of glaucoma are treatable, but macular degeneration is currently not treatable. Diabetes, which is increasing in the population, can also contribute to vision losses (diabetic retinopathy). So about 25% of those at advanced ages (e.g., 80+) are likely to have some degree of visual impairment.

2.1.2 Hearing and Balance

2.1.2.1 Hearing

Whether through cumulative environmental exposure to loud sounds or through genetic influences, many people, particularly men, tend to lose hearing acuity as they enter their 50s. Sounds in the upper frequency range are the most affected. The condition is known as presbycusis. Such losses make it more difficult to process speech sounds, particularly the high-pitched components that enable detection of phonemes such as "s" or "t." Speech sounds that comprise phonemes (basic building blocks), although complex with multiple frequencies, typically have most of their energy in frequency ranges from 500–2,000 Hz. Presbycusis makes speech perception more difficult, particularly in noisy environments. The prevalence of speech-frequency hearing loss in a United States sample can be seen in Figure 2.2.

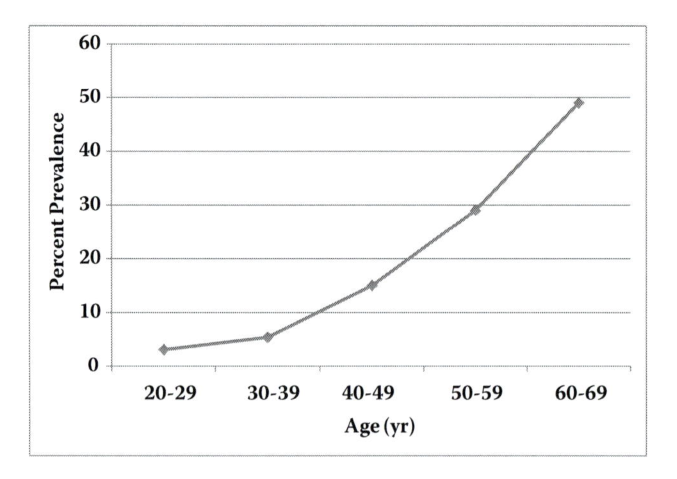

Figure 2.2 United States prevalence of speech-frequency hearing loss by age. (Data from Agrawal, Y., Platz, E.A., & Niparko, J.K., 2008. Prevalence of hearing loss and differences by demographic characteristics among US adults: Data from the National Health and Nutrition Examination Survey, 1999–2004. *Archives of Internal Medicine,* 168, 1522–30.)

In old age, ability to detect some frequencies virtually disappears unless the sounds are highly amplified. As an example, a pure tone with a pitch of 8,000 Hz must be in excess of 90 dB intensity for the average 80-year-old male to detect it. (Exposure to sound at 85 dB over an extended time period is associated with hearing loss in young adulthood.) Much of the hearing loss is attributable to loss of hair cells in the cochlea and later in life to losses in transmission from the auditory nerve through to the auditory cortical centers in the brain, so simple amplification may not help those with neural conduction problems.

2.1.2.2 Balance

The cochlea also contains part of the sensory system responsible for maintaining balance (the semicircular canals and otoliths) by conveying information about position in space (x, y, z planes). Thus, losses in the integrity of structures in the ear–brain system can also affect balance. Balance relies on a complex set of receptors that include the ear and the eye, as well as skin and muscle receptors that provide proprioceptive and kinesthetic information about relative positioning of the limbs to the body core. Older adults rely much more heavily on vision to support balance and are less able to maintain balance in the absence of light. An example is a test where people are asked to stand on one foot with their eyes closed. Typical older adults are unable to maintain their balance that way for more than a few seconds. Many pharmaceuticals can also affect balance and put older adults at even greater risk for falls (psychoactive drugs are particularly problematic).

2.1.3 *Touch/Haptics*

The field of haptics concerns qualities of touch and location (localization to a body part). Haptic senses include both the perceptions that are aroused passively (such as when something comes in contact with an area of skin) and actively. An example of active haptics would be the case of someone exploring an object solely through touch—for instance, trying to find an object in a drawer without sight of the contents or feeling for a pair of spectacles on a nightstand in the dark. Qualities conveyed through the proprioceptive and kinesthetic receptor systems include temperature, vibration, and pain. In general, as people age they show less fine discrimination for localization on the skin. They experience higher thresholds for detecting stimuli conveyed through these sensory channels and also exhibit slower processing of haptic information. Although generally few signals for operating telehealth systems are conveyed through touch or temperature, the ubiquitous mobile phone does offer the option of indicating important states through vibration (buzzing). For someone with hearing impairments, having a redundant haptic channel can be quite helpful. However, there is an age-related decline in sensitivity to high frequency vibration (60 Hz and above), so it would be wise to use haptic signaling only for low frequency vibration, such as 25 Hz signals.

2.2 *Cognition*

Imagine older adults who are meeting with their physicians (perhaps via videoconference) and hearing the physicians discuss their current medical condition, for instance notifying them that they have adult onset diabetes and that they will need to modify their diet and exercise patterns accordingly. Or imagine that they are being instructed on how to carry out a videoconference session with their home health care nurse using their home computer system and a webcam. How well will they comprehend and remember what they are being told? Imagine that their videoconference system malfunctions and they need to find out what went wrong and correct it. All these tasks engage cognitive abilities.

Cognitive abilities coalesce into two interrelated clusters: crystallized abilities and fluid abilities. Crystallized abilities refer to those that depend on acquiring knowledge from one's culture. Typically, tests of information (asking people to answer questions such as "what is the distance between New York and Washington, DC?" and vocabulary (define the word "telemedicine") tap crystallized ability. Thus, all other things being equal, an older adult is more likely than a younger adult to have knowledge about medical conditions and their treatments. However, all other things are not normally equal. Younger adults tend to have more formal education than older adults, and participating in higher education is a very effective way to increase one's knowledge.

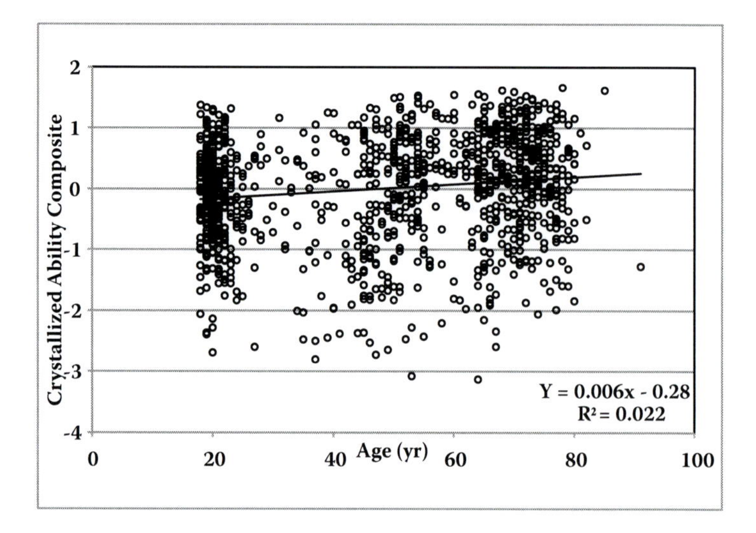

Figure 2.3 Scatterplot of the relationship between crystallized intelligence and chronological age. The sample is a diverse, American sample of ~1,000 people from the Center for Research and Education on Aging and Technology Enhancement (CREATE; www.create-center.org).

Fluid abilities refer to abilities that are relatively knowledge-independent. Capabilities such as speed of processing (measured by a test such as cancel out all the "e's" in this paragraph as quickly as possible), working memory ("spell 'working memory' backwards"), and tests of reasoning ("if all fruits are vegetables and a bear is a fruit, is a bear a vegetable?") typically tap fluid abilities. Normal aging is associated with two different trajectories for these abilities.

Crystallized abilities tend to increase across the lifespan at least through the 60s, whereas fluid abilities tend to decline from the 20s and 30s. The trends for crystallized abilities are shown in Figure 2.3 and fluid abilities in Figure 2.4 using cross-sectional data from a large diverse sample of more than 1,000 people in the Center for Research and Education on Aging and Technology (CREATE) project.

Of course, other variables besides age are important correlates of cognitive abilities. But on balance, older adults will be disadvantaged when having to learn a new procedure compared to younger adults. They typically need about twice as much time to learn new information, though, as pointed out above, they are more likely to have a greater knowledge base than young adults to begin with.

2.2.1 *Speed of Processing*

One of the hallmarks of the aging process is slowing in the rate of information processing. If one looks at how quickly an elementary mental

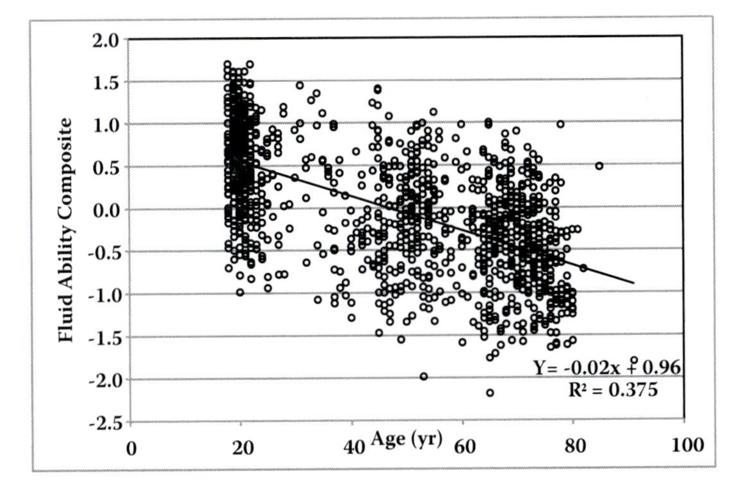

Figure 2.4 Scatterplot of the relationship between fluid intelligence and chronological age. The sample is a diverse, American sample of ~1,000 people from the Center for Research and Education on Aging and Technology Enhancement (CREATE; www.create-center.org).

process occurs, one finds that older adults typically take between 1.5 and 2.0 times as long as younger adults. Motor processing seems to be slowed a bit more than cognitive processes, which in turn are slowed a bit more than perceptual processes. For instance, the time to fixate a word (hold the eye steady and process the word) when reading is only increased by about 10% between ages 20 and 70. However, the time to complete a motor movement may be doubled over that same age interval.

2.2.2 *Attention*

There are multiple aspects of attention. Sustained attention refers to the ability to concentrate and continually monitor some aspect of the environment for the occurrence of a target event. When that target event is not frequent or salient, the task is called a vigilance task. Imagine a nurse monitoring the vital sign equipment for multiple patients. Most of the time the values will stay in normal ranges, but every now and then a critical event may occur. Research shows that vigilance drops pretty quickly over time (declines in performance can be seen after 15 or 20 minutes), but typically, age-related changes in sustained attention are not very large.

Selective attention refers to limited ability to monitor multiple sources of information simultaneously. Typically, an individual can only process information effectively from one channel at a time; for instance, vision but not hearing. If a person has to divide attention across channels (multitask), rapid switching from one channel or task to the other is typically required.

Older adults suffer much greater switching costs than do younger adults. Thus their ability to monitor multiple information sources (e.g., multiple visual locations on a computer screen that indicate current blood pressure, pulse, blood oxygenation) at once will suffer and unless highly experienced, they will perform such tasks much slower than younger adults. A good rule of thumb is to minimize the need to process multiple channels or to identify critical events with warning signals.

2.3 Psychomotor Performance

At some point people must interact physically with telehealth products and systems. That is, they must carry out actions with the equipment. In general, motor control declines with age such that people are less able to carry out precise movements (fine motor control diminishes) and they move much more slowly. Typically, an action that took a younger adult 1 s to carry out would take an older adult 2 s—for instance, when using a mouse to move a cursor to a target location on a computer screen. Some of this decline may represent normal age-related slowing (at the level of brain function), but some may also represent the response to painful arthritic conditions in joints as well as to tremor. One study (n=76) of community-dwelling people in their mid-70s reported that virtually all had at least mild tremor with about a third of the sample experiencing moderate tremor.

One implication is that telehealth systems should not demand quick responding and should adopt time-out functions that are sensible for older users. A good example is the case of typing alphanumeric information on a mobile phone that has a limited input system (nonsmartphones). Typically, the cursor will remain in the same screen position as long as successive button presses occur within the time-out limit. If the person takes longer than expected to respond, the cursor will interpret the next key press on the same button as representing the next character. Research has shown that some phones have too short a time-out function for older adults and hence lead to errors when people attempt to input a character requiring multiple presses on the same key.

Another implication is that fine motor control should not be required to use a device. Miniaturization of devices, while aiding portability, may become a hazard for older adult users. For instance, if a device requires input with finely spaced physical buttons or touch-sensitive icons, older adult users may become frustrated when they accidentally stray onto the wrong button or icon, particularly when they have moderate tremor.

2.4 Anthropometrics

Anthropometrics is a field concerned with measuring a person's physical characteristics such as size, weight, and strength, as well as associated characteristics such as ability to reach and manipulate objects distant from the body (e.g., extent of reach while standing, seated). These dimensions of measurement are used by the design community for manufacturing everything from clothing to seating equipment. The factors that most concern older adults, compared to other segments of the population, are strength, dexterity, and size. People, particularly females, shrink an inch or two (3–5 cm) in height with advanced age and therefore lose reach capability for objects above them. With increased age, strength decreases (e.g., grip strength necessary to open a jar). In addition, the older population is more heavily female than male due to differential mortality by gender (males live about 6 fewer years than females), with women averaging about two-thirds the strength of males given their (average) smaller bones and muscles. Thus telemedicine equipment should be easy to manipulate (e.g., on carts that are easy to wheel), and telemedicine environments such as clinics should be easy to navigate around (e.g., not require excess force to open doors). Further, older men, and particularly older women, are very likely to experience a chronic condition such as arthritis with concomitant difficulty with reaching, grasping, and manipulating objects. Figure 2.5 shows the prevalence of doctor-diagnosed arthritis in the United States for 2007–2009. About 50% of those aged 65+ years will have arthritis, and typically about half of those people will experience significant limitations in functioning. Thus it is critical to choose (and design) equipment with easy to use controls that do not demand much strength, flexibility, or dexterity.

Severe arthritis can also result in disability, wherein older adults have difficulty performing everyday activities, particularly those requiring mobility. Although disability rates associated with increased age had

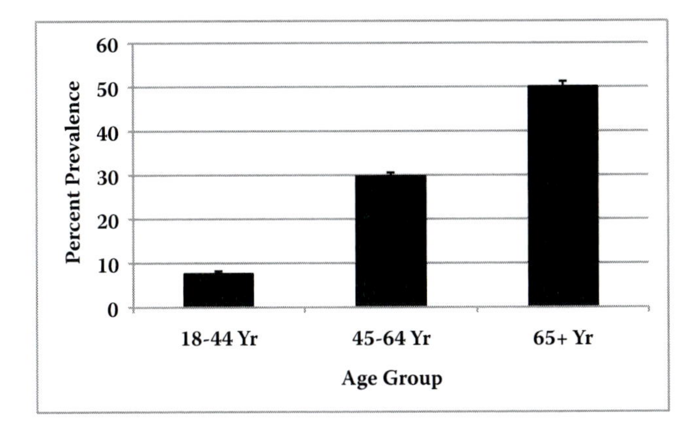

Figure 2.5 Percent prevalence of doctor-diagnosed arthritis in the United States with 95% confidence intervals. (Data from Table 2 of the Centers for Disease Control and Prevention's Morbidity and Mortality Weekly Report, Oct. 8, 2010; http://www.cdc.gov/mmwr/PDF/wk/mm5939.pdf.)

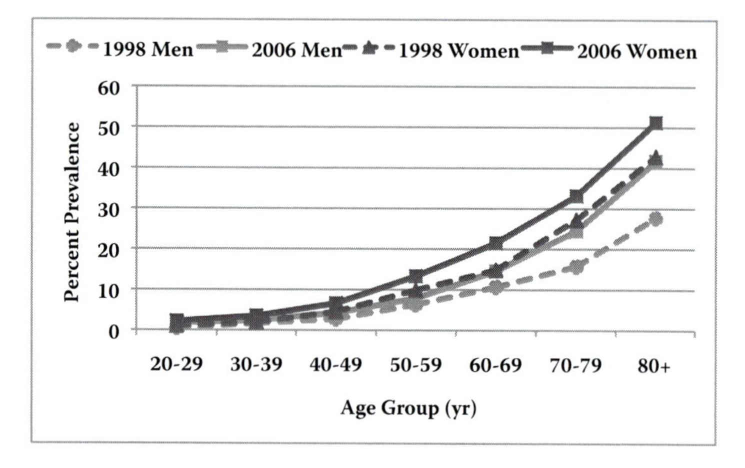

Figure 2.6 United States prevalence of a mobility disability by age and sex. (Crimmins, E.M. & Beltrán-Sánchez, H., 2010. Mortality and morbidity trends: Is there compression of morbidity? *Journal of Gerontology: Social Sciences*, 66B, 1, Table 3, doi:10.1093/geronb/gbq088.)

been declining for the last few decades, some recent United States data suggests that such rates are now increasing, when comparing prevalence rates in 1998 and in 2006, as seen in Figure 2.6. The changes seem most pronounced for the very old.

Providing the opportunity for virtual visits (through videoconferencing) in place of in-person health care visits might help address this trend.

2.5 Attitudes

Attitudes, positive and negative inclinations, for instance, toward telehealth technology, may help or hinder the adoption and use of such technology. Attitudes have been found to be related to factors such as age, education and socioeconomic status, health status and disability, and ethnicity. Not surprisingly, those who are disadvantaged on such factors (older, less educated, lower socioeconomic status (SES), poorer health, more disabled, minority status) tend to have less positive attitudes toward technology in general, and also exhibit lower use. It is not yet clear which of these factors holds primacy in predicting attitudes or use, given that at least one study has shown that cognitive status can be a powerful predictor of technology use. Nonetheless, older adults may be willing to cede some privacy and confidentiality when they understand that, for instance, remote monitoring technology may support their independence.

When considering age in particular, there are strong indications that the value of technology, including health care technology, must be perceived to be strong relative to the costs of adoption. Older adults are more likely than younger adults to weigh benefits more strongly than costs.

Such findings argue for the importance of providing a supportive environment when introducing e-health technology, including providing appropriate training and technical support. This would be true for all users, including health care professionals. Research also indicates that some forms of in-home monitoring are more acceptable than others. For instance, passive monitoring (e.g., through sensors) is rated as more acceptable than cameras in home monitoring systems, at least in certain situations. Nonetheless, older adults are quite willing to trade off confidentiality and privacy for health security when the benefits can be demonstrated to outweigh the risks. However, this willingness to accept monitoring seems restricted to the case of relaying such information to family members or health care providers, but much less so for providing it to government or insurance companies, at least among U.S. seniors.

2.6 Issues of Disability

One risk associated with partitioning capabilities in this way for review (e.g., perception, cognition, attitudes, etc.) is in conveying too fragmented a view of older adult capabilities and also failing to consider trends across time. Comorbidities can increase the risk of activity limitations (disability), though adaptive capabilities can sometimes compensate for ability declines. Figure 2.7 shows the trend across years and age group for the

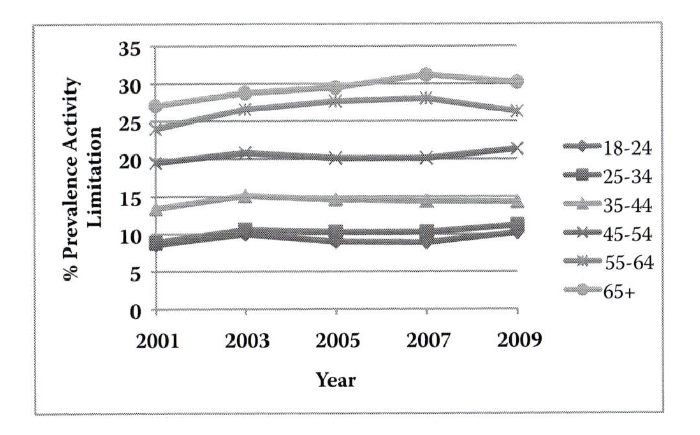

Figure 2.7 Age and time trends for activity limitations in the United States. (Data from the Behavioral Risk Factor Surveillance System, Centers for Disease Control and Prevention. Behavioral Risk Factor Surveillance System Survey Questionnaire. Atlanta, Georgia: U.S. Department of Health and Human Services, Centers for Disease Control and Prevention, 2001–2009. Accessed Feb. 11, 2011, http://apps.nccd.cdc.gov/brfss/age.asp?yr=2001&state=US&qkey=4000&grp=0.)

number of adults in the United States who reported a limitation in activities because of physical, mental, or emotional problems ("Are you limited in any way in any activities because of physical, mental, or emotional problems?").

The bottom line from this Figure is that about 30% of adults aged 65+ consider themselves to be significantly limited due to health-related conditions. After a rising trend since 2001, disability has started to decline for the older age groups, though it may be increasing in younger age groups. It is worth contrasting these trends for the 65+ year-old population with those for mobility disability (Figure 2.6), which showed an increase between 1998 and 2006. Nonetheless, both surveys suggest that attempting to design effective telehealth systems for an aging population is going to be challenging given the "moving target" nature of older adult limitations. Whether the long-term trend is increasing or decreasing for disability (activity limitations) is likely to be a function of the environmental support offered to seniors to enable them to cope successfully with declining abilities.

Perhaps more relevant is a question from the Behavioral Risk Factor Surveillance System (BRFSS) that queries the need to use special equipment to compensate for limitations ("Do you now have any health problem that requires you to use special equipment, such as a cane, a wheelchair, a special bed, or a special telephone?"). Such people are likely to present with mobility limitations that would make a visit to a health professional difficult. Figure 2.8 shows the trends across time and age group in the United States.

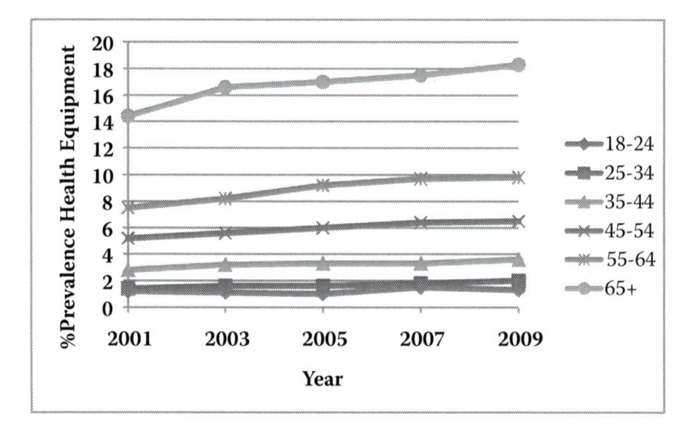

Figure 2.8 Age and time trends for use of health equipment in the United States. (Data from the Behavioral Risk Factor Surveillance System, Centers for Disease Control and Prevention. Behavioral Risk Factor Surveillance System Survey Questionnaire. Atlanta, Georgia: U.S. Department of Health and Human Services, Centers for Disease Control and Prevention, 2001–2009. Accessed Feb. 11, 2011, http://apps.nccd.cdc.gov/brfss/age.asp?yr=2009&state=US&qkey=4001&grp=0.)

The trend here is for a steady increase, particularly for older cohorts, in affirming the use of health equipment. Almost one in five seniors can be expected to make use of "canes, wheelchairs, a special bed or a special telephone." Whether the rise is due to increases in functional decline or increases in availability (perhaps due to increased affordability) for such equipment is not clear. Nonetheless, the data point to the need to be aware of and design for activity limitations that are much more prevalent as people age.

2.7 Recommendations

2.7.1 Guidelines for Vision

Keep the default print size for instructional materials and for text on devices to at least 12 points for fonts if possible. As seen in Figure 2.9, some fonts, such as sans serif Arial, have a greater x-height (the size of a lowercase x character) and should be preferred to others such as Times Roman, a serif font with a smaller x-height.

A useful guideline is to choose an appropriate minimal visual angle for the object to be identified by the viewer. Visual angle is the arctangent of the ratio of the height (and/or width) of the object to its distance from the eye. A good rule of thumb, literally, is that your thumb's width at arm's length subtends a visual angle of about 2 degrees (and thumbnail about 1.6 degrees). Typically you should try to ensure that the object to be identified (say a word on a screen) subtends an angle of at least 0.6 degrees of visual angle at the usual viewing distance for that object.

2.7.2 Guidelines for Hearing

Put warning sounds in the most sensitive frequency band, about 500–1,000 Hz and at least at 60 dB in quiet environments. Augment auditory warnings with visual warnings where possible, or with haptic warnings. The Food and Drug Administration in the United States licenses medical devices and provides some guidelines for testing them to ensure that warnings for devices such as oxygen concentrators are effective.

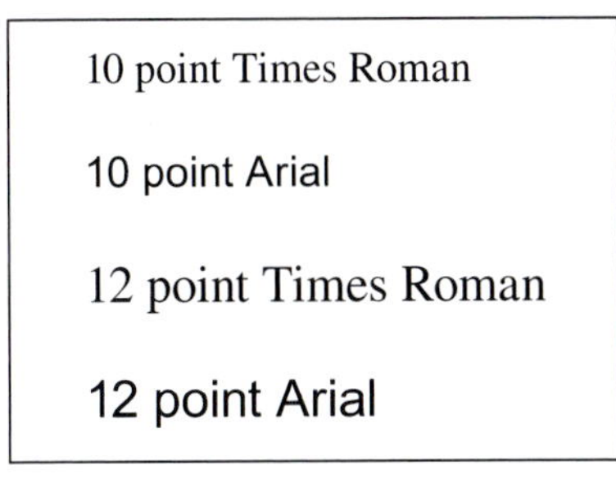

Figure 2.9 An illustration of different fonts and sizes.

2.7.3 Guidelines for Cognition

Ensure adequate time for training older adults to use a new device. A good rule of thumb is to provide twice as much time as that typically allocated for a young adult. Because older adults may have more difficulty focusing attention, ensure that device displays are relatively sparsely populated with only information and try to present just the critical information for performing the task at hand at any one point in a procedure. "Less is more." Similarly, try to minimize the number of steps that must be kept in mind to complete a procedure to avoid taxing working memory capability. If possible, put relevant information in the environment, such as step by step instructions on a sheet of paper.

2.7.4 Guidelines for Motor Performance

Make controls for a device large and easy to manipulate. Keep adequate space between buttons for a control device and ensure that button labels are easy to read. Try to ensure that movement distances are relatively short and that the target locations for those movements are relatively large and easy to access. If repetitive presses are needed to trigger an action, allow adequate time to repeat the button press.

2.7.5 Guidelines for Attitudes

Provide evidence for the benefits of a health care intervention. Ensure that training is sensitive to learning costs that older adults incur by ensuring that training is matched to prior knowledge. If possible, provide self-paced training.

2.8 Suggested Readings

Crimmins, E.M. & Beltrán-Sánchez, H. (2010). Mortality and morbidity trends: Is there compression of morbidity? *Journal of Gerontology: Social Sciences*, 66B, 1, 75–86, doi:10.1093/geronb/gbq088.

Fisk, A.D., Rogers, W.A., Charness, N., Czaja, S.J., & Sharit, J. (2009). *Designing for Older Adults: Principles and Creative Human Factors Approaches*, 2nd ed. Boca Raton: CRC Press.

Jastrzembski, T.S. & Charness, N. (2007). The Model Human Processor and the older adult: Parameter estimation and validation within a mobile phone task. *Journal of Experimental Psychology: Applied*, 13, 224–248.

Kroemer, K.H.E. (2005). *"Extra-Ordinary" Ergonomics: How to Accommodate Small and Big Persons, The Disabled and Elderly, Expectant Mothers, and Children*. Boca Raton: CRC Press.

Steenbekkers, L.P.A. & van Beijsterveldt, C.E.M. (eds.) (1998). *Design-Relevant Characteristics of Aging Users*. Delft, The Netherlands: Delft University Press.

chapter 3

Health Care Environments and Their Characteristics

In this chapter we summarize some of the trends for where health care is delivered and focus on design issues for telemedicine clinic facilities. We also outline some of the critical detection issues involved in home monitoring systems.

People started seeking health care in hospital settings in North America with much greater frequency in the 1940s. For instance, in the prior century women gave birth to children at home, and this activity shifted to the hospital. Similarly, people died at home most of the time, and also that shifted to hospitals. Although the latter trend has reversed somewhat for deaths, in part due to the development of hospice care, the former trend has persisted for childbirth. Similarly, it was much more common to have physicians visit patients at home in the 1940s and 1950s than it is today when the usual visit is a patient to a physician's office. Although telehealth holds out the promise that people will have to travel less to access health care, it is still the case that telehealth often routes information through hospitals and clinics. In fact, videoconferencing with specialists often consists of a hospital venue on one end (with a specialist) and a remote clinic on the other (with the client).

3.1 Telemedicine Clinic Design

When designing a facility for telemedicine, there are several things to consider from a human factors point of view as well as from a practicality point of view. If the facility is likely to serve older patients, there are a few additional design aspects to consider. The first thing to realize is that most telemedicine clinics are not going to be newly designed and built. In all likelihood they will be existing rooms converted to telemedicine clinic rooms. Quite often the former room will not even have been used for clinical purposes, but may have simply been a storage area cleared out for telemedicine use. Therefore, design is often a challenge, but there are a few basic principles that can be followed to create a workable clinical space.

3.1.1 Start with a Plan

When planning a facility, it is useful to start out by measuring the space and drawing out a floor plan to indicate where the lighting fixtures go, where the doors and windows are, where the air vents are, and so on. It also helps to have the people who are going to use the room think about and possibly act out the various scenarios likely to occur in the room. For example, rheumatology clinics often see a greater number of older patients than younger ones. A key part of many rheumatology exams is assessment of gait and the patient's ability to navigate from one location to another. In telemedicine the consulting rheumatologist needs to remotely view the patient walking from one end of a room to the other using real-time videoconferencing equipment. The clinic room therefore needs to be long enough to accommodate this walk, free of obstacles to avoid tripping and falling, and possibly roomy enough to accommodate walkers. The camera needs to either be remotely moved by the telerheumatologist to follow the patient or the onsite health care provider needs to be able to move it.

3.1.2 Placing the Equipment

Most telemedicine clinic rooms are designed to accommodate both real-time video equipment as well as store-and-forward equipment. The actual design of course depends on the designated room and the operation requirements, but at a minimum it needs to be able to accommodate all the equipment and two people comfortably—the patient and the health care provider. There should be a desk with a computer that will likely serve as the store-and-forward hub where images can be transferred from digital cameras, case records created, and data transmitted to the teleconsultant for interpretation. A fax machine on the desk is useful because additional information is often faxed for cases and having it colocated with the computer improves efficiency. A telephone should also be on the desk so the referring and consulting health care providers can easily communicate while viewing information on the computer. The key is to have all the necessary equipment organized with easy reaching distance so the site coordinator and health care providers do not risk injury trying to access and use the equipment. Standard ergonomic concerns about monitor height, monitor distance, mouse placement, and task lighting should be observed (OSHA, 2010).

The rest of the telemedicine equipment (e.g., video unit, peripheral devices such as electronic stethoscopes, digital cameras with their docking stations) needs to be strategically placed as well. The room cannot be too crowded, and there cannot be lots of wires hanging loose or running along the floor. This is especially crucial for older patients, who may have mobility and stability problems. Someone with a cane, walker, or wheelchair needs to be able to enter the room and navigate around it safely without worrying about tripping on loose wires, bumping into furniture/equipment, or injuring themselves.

3.1.3 *Room Location*

The geographic location of the room is also very important. For example, if the room is stationed near the out-patient check-in wing of a hospital or clinic there will likely be a wide variety of cases referred to telemedicine simply by proximity and familiarity. A room in the pediatric wing will yield more pediatric cases, but the overall practice may suffer because it is too difficult to send patients to a dedicated wing. One option is to have a dedicated telemedicine room but also have equipment that is portable and easy to manipulate so it can be transported to the patient. For something like dermatology this is quite feasible, as the key piece of equipment is a digital camera and perhaps dedicated task lighting. Likewise it is often impractical to transport a cardiology patient to the telemedicine equipment, but there are portable EKG devices that can be taken to the patient. Even real-time video devices are becoming quite portable (some are even robotically driven, like the InTouch system, and can easily be transported around hospitals and clinics for real-time teleconsults). These types of portable devices are extremely useful for older patients as it relieves the burden of them having to walk from one area of the hospital to another. It also saves time, as older patients tend to be slower getting from place to place.

3.1.4 *Environmental Considerations*

Room environment is also something to consider because many sites (both urban and rural) have environmental issues. For example, fine dirt or dust blown in from the outside can ruin equipment and cause problems for patients. As older patients often have respiratory problems, it is necessary to ensure that the telemedicine room is as dust and dirt free as possible—especially if it is a nonclinical room converted to be used as a clinical room. Dust filters may be required for the air system. Heat can be a big problem because of the size of the room and the amount of electronic equipment stored and used. Aside from protecting the equipment, the patient needs to be protected as well. Patients who are already not feeling well or are stressed by being in a hospital may react poorly if placed in a small, hot room for even a short amount of time. Dedicated fans may be needed to keep the equipment and general room environment cool. If humidity is an issue, dehumidifiers may be needed to protect equipment.

3.1.5 Lighting in the Telemedicine Room

Lighting is a crucial design issue that is often overlooked but really needs to be considered carefully. A telemedicine room will likely serve many purposes, so a single lighting system may not suffice. At times the room will simply serve as an office in which the site coordinator or health care provider works on patient records or other paperwork. In this case, standard OSHA guidelines for office lighting for computer environments should be used. Brighter lights may be needed when a patient is present in the room, at least initially. This may be particularly important for older patients with degraded vision to avoid them tripping or bumping into things and risking injury. Light levels for older adults generally need to be about 50% over those comfortable for younger people (this aids their color perception as well), though one needs to be careful to avoid glare (for instance, by using matte surfaces).

In the clinical environment good lighting is critical. It is probably easier to establish a trusting relationship if the patient is comfortable and is not straining to see the health care provider and the rest of (what is likely a strange, technology-filled) environment. If the health care provider is going to show older patients something such as the label on a medication, the color of some pills, radiographic images, or some other data, it is important that the patients be able to clearly see the information so they can better comprehend it.

Once an exam is taking place or images are being acquired for the telemedicine consult, the room lighting can be adjusted as appropriate. For example, to acquire teledermatology and other images with a still digital camera, the room should be well lit (150 ft candles), preferably using light sources as close to white light as possible. Instead of incandescent lights, fluorescent daylight or full-spectrum bulbs should be used. Task lighting may be useful in these types of situations. For real-time video teleconsults, lighting is best between 300–500 lux and should be directed at an angle to the participants, so it may be necessary to buy fixtures on a pole to direct light where it is needed. The key in telemedicine is that the teleconsult participants at both ends need to clearly see each other, and the participants need to look as close to "normal" as possible with respect to skin tone, etc., because these are diagnostic encounters.

3.1.6 Other Room Design Considerations

The room background (e.g., walls, floors) is critical as well. Light blue is the recommended color for telemedicine rooms, and it is recommended that one or two walls be painted blue but not the whole room. This way the color temperature of the skin will not be affected—people will not look bluer than they would naturally. Flat latex blue paint is preferred over gloss or semigloss to avoid glare and reflections (even though glossy paints are preferred in hospitals because they are easier to clean). Glare is especially hard on older patients who already have vision problems.

It is also important to keep the camera view as uncluttered as possible on both sides of a teleconference meeting. From the patient's perspective, they want to be able to focus on the teleclinician without distracting details or objects in the background. This is especially true for older patients whose vision is likely less than optimal; if they are straining to figure out what is in the background, they may be distracted from the diagnostic session. Likewise, the teleclinician needs to have an unobstructed view of the patient without a lot of clutter so they do not get distracted.

3.1.7 *Video and Audio Issues*

There are also a few other concerns for real-time teleconferencing when the patient is an older adult. It is important to think about what size the monitor screen is for viewing the teleclinician. In most cases the camera aimed at the patient needs to be at least 5 feet away from him or her to capture the most information possible (i.e., head as well as full body shots), and in general the camera is placed on top of the monitor used for viewing the teleconsultant. At this distance the older patient may have trouble seeing the image of the teleconsultant if the screen is too small. Larger screens (50 inch) are desirable as long as the resolution is adequate. High-definition cameras and displays are quickly becoming the standard, so if possible these should be used to help compensate for the poorer vision of older patients.

The speaker and microphone capabilities and placement are also an issue. Because older patients are often soft-spoken or have trouble projecting, the microphone needs to be placed closer to them perhaps than with younger patients. The speakers may either have to be placed closer or the volume turned up so as to compensate for hearing loss in the older patient. It is important in all situations to ask the patient at the beginning of the teleconsult if they are able to see and hear the teleclinician comfortably and make adjustments if necessary.

3.2 *Homes*

Because of the high cost of providing health care in hospitals in particular and in doctor's offices and clinics in general, many insurers of health care services are looking to telehealth as a means of lowering their costs. It should be remembered that the main reason that health care moved from the home to the hospital in the first place was to provide a better environment for health care service delivery. Given the enormous variability in home environments compared to those found in the office, the clinic, or the hospital, telehomecare must meet many challenges. Resources that can be taken for granted in formal health care settings, such as electrical power, Internet access, and even lighting may not be as readily available or reliable in the home.

3.2.1 Connectivity

Telemedicine requires communication networks and electrical power. Except for remote rural locales, electrical power can be assumed to be present. (However, in many American inner cities, for residents who are unable to pay, electrical services may be turned off and might have to be subsidized to enable some types of telehealth installations.) The earliest and still most important remote access point in the home is the telephone, which was at nearly 98% penetration rates in the United States in 2008 (counting both wired and wireless connections). However, there has been a dramatic shift in the type of telephones in use since the advent of the mobile phone. Wired phone utilization rates appear to be dropping in homes in general, as people rely more on mobile phones. (In many developing countries mobile phones have become the main communication channel.) About 20% of U.S. households were solely mobile phone users in 2008.

Given their generally slower rate of technology adoption, older adult households are more likely to have a wired connection and less likely to have a mobile phone present as well. Whereas 41.5% of 25–29 year olds lived in wireless-only households, only about 3.3% of those 65+ did. A 2008 Pew Internet and American Life survey showed that 70% of 65–74 year olds owned mobile phones, 50% of 75–84 year olds, and 30% of 85+ year olds. However, future cohorts of older adults will more closely resemble today's younger adult mobile phone users. Figure 3.1 shows the trends for living in wireless-only households in the United States. Future cohorts of older adults are much less likely to have wired connections in their households than today's older cohorts.

One positive trend for telehealth is the increased adoption of broadband for Internet access in many countries at speeds that can support effective videoconferencing. In general, older adults are less likely to use the Internet than younger adults and less likely to have broadband access as well. The age differential in use of the Internet can be seen in Figure 3.2, which shows the trend across time for the United States by age group.

The good news is the trend for older adults to show the greatest percent increase of all age groups. The bad news is that they started from a very low adoption rate and the majority of those aged 65+ still do not use the Internet. Also, these are not longitudinal data. Data are from repeated cross-sectional surveys, so some of the improvement probably stems from 50- to 64-year-old computer or Internet users in 1995 migrating into the 65+ year-old cohort in 2010.

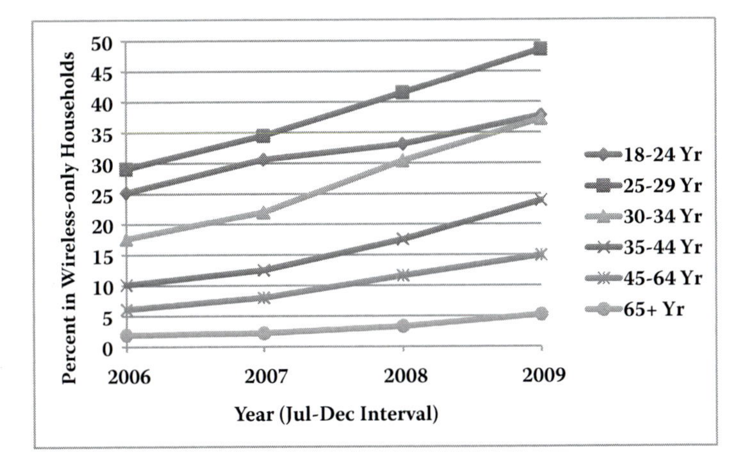

Figure 3.1 Percent living in wireless-only households by age group, United States. (Data is from Table 2 in the Centers for Disease Control and Prevention's report from the National Health Interview Survey early release publication, http://www.cdc.gov/nchs/data/nhis/earlyrelease/wireless201005.htm.)

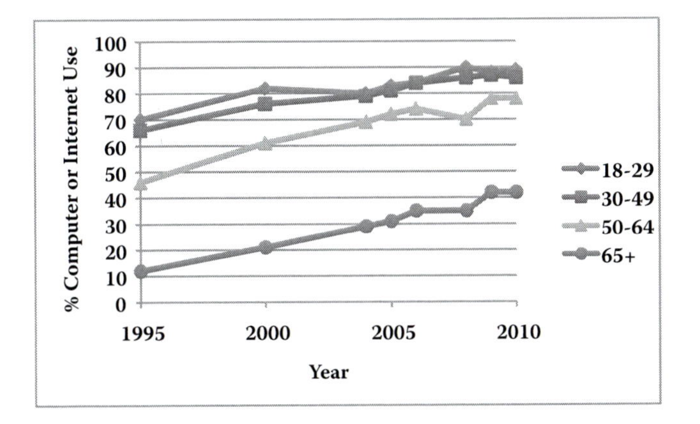

Figure 3.2 Percent computer or Internet use by age group and year in the United States. (Data accessed March 11, 2011, http://www.census.gov/compendia/statab/2011/tables/11s1157.xls.)

There are a number of important implications from this figure. First, expecting older adults to access information from a health care website is not realistic, unless both equipment and training is provided. Second, personal electronic health record software is not likely to be of immediate use to many seniors. In short, the majority of today's seniors may need to rely on friends or family members to help them access the Internet.

The figures are even less encouraging when looking at Internet use worldwide. For instance, in the UK, a developed nation, about 16% of those aged 65+ had used the Internet in the month of April in 2007 (http://www.census.gov/prod/2009pubs/p95-09-1.pdf, accessed 3/14/11). The International Telecommunications Union reported that in 2010 about 30% of people around the world were Internet users (http://www.itu.int/ITU-D/ict/statistics/at_glance/KeyTelecom.html, accessed 3/14/11). Use varies with region, with a low of 10% in Africa and a high of 65% in Europe. About 8% of world users have fixed broadband connections and 14% have mobile broadband connections. However, senior users would likely be a very small percentage of all users.

However, access to the Internet, particularly with broadband, is increasing, and many countries are undertaking significant initiatives to improve such access. For instance, in 2010 Finland mandated home access to a broadband connection as a right of citizenship. In a relatively short time frame households in the United States have moved from phone line Internet access to broadband sources such as television cable lines and DSL for wired phone lines. And as has been noted in some U.S. surveys, ethnic minorities such as African-Americans, who tend to have much lower broadband access, are more likely to access the Internet through a mobile phone than from a home computer. Many new telehealth applications are being developed to take advantage of mobile phone and tablet technology. This trend will be of particular benefit to developing countries that are building wireless-only telecommunications infrastructures.

Another positive development is that many consumers who do have home Internet access set up networks via wireless routers that allow multiple devices to share a single Internet connection. Again, older households tend to lag in this respect. Further, even when a network is running in an older adult's household, it is often difficult to interact with, given that older residents in particular are less likely to be knowledgeable about it (e.g., know passwords for accessing a router). Often the network has been set up for them by relatives or by a computer store. Further, the resident will be concerned about any changes made to accommodate new equipment. The authors have seen examples such as one case where an older adult who had consented to be in a telehealth study (and who was to be financially compensated for participating), withdrew consent once he saw that his system was going to be modified. Significant technical support will need to be provided by the installer when anything goes wrong, including things that are unlikely to be the fault of the telehealth provider.

One possibility to avoid disrupting existing home networks is to take advantage of developing mobile phone networks to carry telehealth data, particularly given the increases in bandwidth being rolled out by mobile phone providers (so-called 3G and 4G networks) either by using mobile phones to transmit data or by using equipment with cellular modems.

3.2.2 Lighting

Particularly in the case of videoconferencing, having adequate lighting is important for ensuring communication effectiveness. Unlike the case of hospital or clinic environments, where building codes and practices typically follow lighting standards (e.g., IES, http://www.iesna.org/), home environments in North America have no luminance requirements. As a result, average luminance levels (more specifically, reflectance measured from white pages in books, newspapers) can be quite low, much less than the typical 100 cd/m^2 found in hospital and business environments. A study of Tallahassee, Florida, homes found average light levels of 30 cd/m^2. In one trailer home there was only a single 40 W bulb present. Hence we recommend ensuring that webcams or videoconferencing cameras work well in low light conditions, or that supplemental luminaires (light sources) be provided to the homeowner (positioned to ensure that lighting is stronger in front of than behind the person).

3.3 Suggested Readings

Krupinski, E.A., Burdick, A., Pak, H., et al. (2008). American Telemedicine Association's practice guidelines for teledermatology. *Telemed & eHealth,* 14,289–302.

Occupational Safety & Health Administration (OSHA). (2010). Computer workstations. Retrieved from http://www.osha.gov/SLTC/etools/computerworkstations/ (accessed 3/11/11).

chapter 4

Telemedicine Fields and Human Factors Issues

In this chapter we review some of the major specialties within telemedicine and provide practical advice about ways to improve remote health care delivery.

4.1 Teleradiology

With teleradiology as with most other clinical specialties, there are two sides of the equation—the patient and the radiologist. It is different from other clinical specialties, however, in the sense that the radiologist and patient never (or very rarely) meet. The same is true with conventional radiology as well, except for interventional procedures where the radiologist does interact with the patient. Interventional radiology (e.g., balloon angioplasty, line/tube insertion, angiography, and other image-guided minimally invasive procedures) to date, however, has yet to be done in the context of teleradiology, for obvious reasons.

4.1.1 Teleradiology and Older Patients

For the patient side of the equation, the person(s) interacting with the patient is typically the radiology technologist, and therefore it is the technologist that needs to be particularly aware of issues that arise when older patients have radiographic exams. Older patients, especially those with mobility disabilities (e.g., walking aids), will require extra help climbing onto the examination table, sitting up after the exam is acquired (due to the lack of handholds and the surface pad not being fixed in place), and maintaining position if the table moves (e.g., during a fluoroscopic exam where the table moves from horizontal to vertical). Although the core image acquisition technology cannot really be changed or adjusted specifically for older patients, there are easy steps that can be taken such as replacing the stepstool to get on the table with a more rugged one that has hand rails and manually helping the patient get onto and off of the table. It is also useful for a radiology department to keep a standard walker on the premises for those patients who do not typically use a walker but might need the added support.

Balance and stability issues in general are a consideration with older patients, and requiring them to climb on and off high exam tables can result in more falls than simply navigating from room to room. Balance and stability problems can be further compounded in older adults because they are often on a variety of medications that can affect these capabilities. Older patients also may need extra time during exam preparation because of slowness in changing clothes and moving from one room to the next, especially if they have added constraints such as oxygen or walking aids. It may be useful to add a little extra time into the imaging schedule if it is known that a patient is an older adult.

Older patients often have other disabilities that should be considered during the imaging procedure as well. For example, patients with strokes are often mobility-constrained and require a significant amount of help getting from one location or position to another. It is important for the technologist to help the patients move rather than dragging them or forcing them into required positions. If patients are pulled by their arms they could suffer joint or nerve damage. For the technologist it is also important not to let the patient hang on to his or her neck while being helped, as this could injure the technologist. Getting extra help is often the easiest and safest way to avoid injuries while moving patients in the acquisition room.

The technologist (and the radiologist) needs to be aware of any prosthetic devices, implants, pacemakers, or other devices that cannot be removed during image acquisition as they may cause artifacts or contraindicate CT or MRI exams. It is also important to carefully consider imaging instructions and their delivery (e.g., when to hold their breath and for how long), as many patients may have diminished eyesight, hearing, and mental capacity. To reduce anxiety due to confusion or misunderstanding, it is often useful to have the patient's caretaker involved as much as possible. Clearly they will not be allowed in the x-ray room during image acquisition for safety reasons, but they can be kept close to the technologist in the protected area where the patient can see them for reassurance if the facility permits this. Overall, the best thing the technologist can do with older patients is communicate, explaining step by step throughout the procedure what is required of the patient and exactly what the technologist is doing at every step along the way.

4.1.2 Issues for the Teleradiologist

For the radiologist interpreting the exam, there are other issues to consider. In many cases older patients are not able to provide adequate clinical information (e.g., last time they were imaged, what the exact symptoms are, how long the symptoms have been present), so the radiologist has no a priori knowledge about why the exam has been acquired. Another problem is that there are really very few standards with respect to what is normal in an older patient. It is often difficult to distinguish normal manifestations of old age from pathological changes. Common diseases often exhibit different characteristics in older than in younger patients, confounding the problem even further (e.g., pneumonia is characterized by segmental air-space opacity in younger but as patchy infiltrate in older adults). One solution is to use advanced technologies such as CT or MRI instead of plain x-ray techniques, although there are increased costs associated with these exams. Many of these more advanced techniques, however, utilize contrast agents, and older adults are often more susceptible to contrast reactions than younger people, so this too needs to be considered.

Another aspect to consider is what happens as radiologists grow older. Radiology is a vision-based specialty. Images need to be viewed and interpreted diagnostically. If the vision of the radiologist is impaired it could significantly impact his or her ability to accurately interpret images. For example, although it is generally recommended that people get their eyes checked annually (especially for individuals with vision problems or who wear corrective lenses), radiologists get their eyes examined closer to every two years. It is also important to keep in mind that as people get older the eyes generally need to work harder to accommodate (i.e., maintain focus). Again, given that radiology is a vision-based specialty, it is important that radiologists be able to maintain proper focus on the display to optimize their ability to detect abnormalities. Older radiologists have significantly reduced ability to maintain accommodative focus as the day progresses, and they spend more time reading images compared to younger residents. As radiologists get older themselves they need to monitor their eyesight in general through regular exams as well as monitor their daily levels of visual fatigue as this may lead to increased error rates.

4.2 Telepathology

Telepathology is very similar to radiology in that the pathologist and the patient rarely interact. As pathology is a vision-based specialty like radiology, the same concerns raised above for teleradiology apply here as well. Pathologists should have their vision checked on a regular basis, and they should monitor their visual fatigue levels as the working day progresses so as to avoid risking errors due to fatigue and distraction. Pathologists also need to familiarize themselves with the differences between normal aging and pathological processes. Thus it is important for the pathologist to receive as much clinical information (e.g., age, gender, existing conditions) as possible about the patient so they have some a priori information to rely on when interpreting the specimen data.

4.2.1 Acquiring Pathology Samples and the Patient

From the patient's perspective, the acquisition of the sample (e.g., tissue, sputum) is the key event, and the health care specialist acquiring those samples may need to consider some important issues with older patients. Again, communication is the key step in a successful pathology procedure as it was with radiology. The clinician needs to ensure that the older adults understand why the sample is being acquired, what the steps are, what they can expect to feel (especially if some pain might be involved), and what is required in terms of follow-up (e.g., if a biopsy of the skin is taken, how long should it remain covered, and how long will it take to heal). Reducing anxiety and the potential for misunderstanding is crucial. If it is possible to involve the patient's caretaker in the procedure, this should be considered (e.g., present in the room, holding their hand). Although the data are mixed, there is some evidence that pain thresholds and perceptions differ as a function of age, gender, and cognitive functioning, so it may be important for the clinician acquiring samples to be aware of this fact and ask about pain experience during procedures that have the potential to cause pain.

4.3 Teledermatology

4.3.1 Modes of Conducting Teledermatology Consults

There are two modes in which teledermatology consults take place—real time using videoconferencing technology and store and forward using digital photographs and other electronic data. Both typically involve patients visiting their local health care provider and being seen by the dermatology specialist at a distance. One of the main advantages of teledermatology is the reduction in travel required for the patient to see the specialty dermatologist. This can be especially beneficial to older patients who cannot drive, cannot drive long distances, or have limited access to transportation in general. With teledermatology, the patients visit their local health care provider, which is often much easier and has less impact on their regular routine.

4.3.2 What the Patient Needs to Know about Teledermatology

In this case there are really three perspectives that need to be taken into account: the patient's, the local health care provider's, and the teledermatologist's. For both real-time and store-and-forward consultations, the patient needs to be educated with respect to the technology (e.g., video or digital still camera, microphones, speakers, monitors); what security measures are being taken to preserve patient information and confidentiality;

the goals of the consultation; the timeframe involved (especially with store and forward, as the consult is asynchronous with the local office visit); the roles of the local referring and distant consulting clinicians (i.e., who is the person ultimately responsible for their care); and what their options are if they do not want to be involved in a teleconsult. They should also be informed about the limitations of the consultation (e.g., the teledermatologist cannot examine by touch).

For real-time sessions, the patients should first be given a short lesson on where to look (i.e., where the camera is) and where to speak (i.e., where the microphone is). For older patients this is important because they may have vision problems and therefore their distance from the camera and viewing monitor may need to be adjusted to account for vision limitations. It may also be necessary to adjust the volume of the speakers so older patients with hearing limitations can adequately hear the teledermatologist. The microphones may need to be placed closer or the sensitivity adjusted as older adults' voices may be softer (less able to project) than those of younger patients.

4.3.3 *What the Clinician Needs to Know*

Both the local clinician and teledermatologist should keep in mind that it may be necessary to remind the patient about where to look, etc., during the encounter, as older patients might have trouble remembering instructions. The local health care provider may need to use a handheld exam camera to acquire images for the teledermatologist to view, as older patients may have trouble standing up and showing relevant body areas to the main camera. When using the handheld camera, the local health care provider should carefully position the patients so they are comfortable and able to maintain that position without moving a lot (to avoid blurred images) for a few minutes at a time so the teledermatologist can carefully examine the images. The local health care providers need to be aware that they are likely going to have to repeat any recommendations made during the real-time session after it is over and likely provide a written version of recommendations and instructions to older patients in case memory could be a problem.

For store-and-forward teleconsultations, the local health care provider typically acquires photographs of the affected areas of the body for transmission to the teledermatologist. Again, the image acquisition process, privacy measures, and so on need to be fully explained to the patient. As with the real-time exam camera, the local health care provider should carefully position the patients so they are comfortable and able to maintain that position without moving a lot (to avoid blurred images) for a few minutes at a time so the digital still images can be acquired with good quality. For both real-time and store-and-forward consultations, it may be necessary to photograph sensitive areas of the body (e.g., genitals), and older patients may be much less willing to have these areas photographed than younger patients. The need for these images must be carefully explained to the patients and the security measures may need to be reiterated.

Balance and stability issues come into play in dermatology consults as well, depending on where the region of interest to be photographed is. For example, younger patients may be readily able to lift their foot for a photograph of the underside of the foot, but an older person will more likely need to be seated and possibly require help lifting the foot, turning it properly, and holding it steady for the photography. The local health care provider needs to be able to help the patient as well as acquire the photographs. A simple way to avoid problems is to get help so one person acquires the images while the other helps the patient.

Teledermatologists in a real-time consultation need to be aware of the physical (vision and hearing primarily) and cognitive limitations of older patients. As with any other clinical specialty, the more background information available about the problem the better. With dermatology, such issues as when the problem first arose, how long has it been present, has it happened before, and what medications were used to treat it are all very important, but older patients may be less able to recall and provide accurate details about these issues than a younger patient. In this case the local health care provider may be able to provide some information from the patient record, but both the referring and consulting clinicians have to realize that they may not be able to get all the desired information.

4.3.4 Some Technical Issues

The teledermatologist (and the local health care provider) also need to be aware of the basic changes that occur with aging skin and be able to differentiate normal aging processes from pathological conditions. Older skin tends to have more sun damage, be more wrinkled, have more normal discolorations (i.e., irregular pigmentations), and have more benign conditions (e.g., skin tags) than younger patients. For the health care provider acquiring the images, it may be necessary to adjust the photography or acquire more images of the same location from different angles to capture a good reference range of these various normal background features. It may be necessary to spread wrinkled skin flatter to fully expose a potential lesion of interest. Lighting conditions may need to be adjusted to better illuminate the skin. The teledermatologist needs to be informed about any unusual steps that were taken to acquire the images, especially for store-and-forward consultations. It is also important with a store-and-forward consultation (maybe more so than with real-time) that the local health care provider follow up with the patient once the teledermatologist provides the consult. Typically a teledermatologist gets the report back to the local clinician within a reasonably short amount of time (24–48 hours), but even in that case the patient has obviously left the clinic. The local provider needs to contact the patient directly to convey the results and provide recommendations. This is especially true for older adults, where anxiety about the results, treatment options, etc., may be higher than in younger patients. With respect to treatment, the teledermatologist needs to realize as well that older patients do not always react the same way to medications as younger patients and should inform the local health care provider about these differences and what to look for.

4.4 Teleophthalmology

Currently the most common teleophthalmology consultations are diabetic retinopathy screening exams. For the most part, teleophthalmology is a store-and-forward application in which the images of the eye are acquired using specialized ophthalmology equipment (e.g., nonmydriatic digital camera) that is used in traditional practice as well as the teleapplication. Users of the technology for acquiring diabetic retinopathy screening images are generally trained specifically on the operation of the equipment, but if dealing with an older clientele, they should be aware of a few additional considerations as well. Older patients (especially those with a preexisting condition such as diabetes, which affects a variety of physiological systems) are subject to a wider variety of vision problems than younger patients (even those with diabetes).

4.4.1 Patients and Teleophthalmology

Older patients are more likely to have glaucoma, cataracts, macular degeneration, and general age-related disorders compared to younger patients. Thus, the person acquiring the images needs to be aware that these conditions might exist and may need to adapt the imaging sequences and possibly the number of images to acquire sufficient data for the teleophthalmologist. This person therefore needs to be able to communicate with the patient to find out if there are any preexisting vision conditions and be able to recognize their presence during the exam if the patient is unaware of their existence.

4.4.2 Acquiring and Interpreting Teleophthalmology Images

As with other specialties, the person interacting with older patients needs to be aware of potential cognitive decline that may impair the patient's ability to remember the exact nature of the conditions, what medications they are taking, and how long and what severity of symptoms have been present. Older patients may be even more frustrated with general age-related declines in vision than with other age-related declines because humans rely so much on vision in nearly every situation and circumstance. The patient may not even be able to differentiate normal decline with more severe disorders, so communication and recording of the nature of the problems for the teleophthalmologist is crucial compared to the patient interacting with the ophthalmologist directly.

In general, it is important for the local person acquiring the images to be aware of general limitations of older patients. As with other imaging specialties, the patient needs to sit still while the images are being acquired, and older patients may find it difficult to stay still for prolonged periods of time. If there are numerous images to be acquired, it may be necessary to space them apart to let the patient rest a bit between acquisitions. Older patients may also have trouble keeping their head pressed again the chinrest/headrest effectively, so they may need someone to hold their head, or a strap could be considered. If the exam requires dilation of the eye, it is important to consider that this represents potentially a compounding (although temporary) disability for the older patients, who may already have vision, balance, and stability issues. It may be necessary to keep older patients in the clinic longer and monitor their progress after the exam until the dilation wears off.

For the teleophthalmologist it is likewise crucial to have as much information as possible available about the patient (e.g., age, gender, history of conditions, current problems). Teleophthalmology is for the most part a store-and-forward application; if information is not available when they view the images, it is not easy to get more information because the patient is no longer at the referring site. As with other subspecialties, the teleophthalmologist needs to be aware of normal changes in the appearance of older adults' eyes as opposed to pathological changes, to render accurate diagnoses. As with store-and-forward teledermatology, it is important for the local health care provider and the teleophthalmologist to get the results and recommendations back to the patient as quickly as possible and with as much additional information as possible to ensure that the older patient understands the results and what needs to be done.

4.5 Telesurgery

Telesurgery is really still in its infancy, although there are more and more applications evolving. It is likely that with telesurgery, more than other teleapplications, the older patient may need to be assured more strongly than with younger patients that it is indeed safe to be operated on at a distance. Meetings with the surgeon (most likely using real-time videoconferencing) should take place prior to and after the surgery to explain the procedures, technology, possible complications, postsurgery procedures, and so on to the patient. As there has been very little research on this topic, however, it is difficult to predict. There are, however, certain issues that should be considered with older patients and telesurgery once it does become more widespread.

4.5.1 *Anesthesia and Older Adults*

One concern is the anesthesia. Older patients need to be evaluated prior to receiving anesthesia regarding their mental status, cardiac conditions, pulmonary conditions, level of frailty, whether they are dehydrated, what medications they are on, and history of prior surgeries and reactions. With telesurgery these concerns are even greater than with in-person surgery because although the anesthesiologist is likely onsite, the surgeon is remote and his or her attention may be more on the surgical tasks at hand than on the general remote environment. Thus they may be less aware of the patient status than if they were there in person and may need to rely more on the attention and feedback of those actually present to monitor the patient's status.

Older patients are also more sensitive to anesthetic agents (i.e., require less to achieve desired outcomes) and often require more time to recover completely. Given that the telesurgeon is likely to "log off" after the surgery, the burden of monitoring the patient after the procedure is on the local health care providers, so they need to be aware of differences in recovery time with older patients. This is especially true with outpatient surgeries where the patient is sent home after the procedure. Older patients should likely be kept on premises longer than younger patients. Again, those patients with mobility, balance, or stability issues will need closer monitoring than those without these added factors.

4.5.2 *Surgeon Training with Robotic Devices*

From the perspective of the telesurgeons, the key human factors consideration is training with the robotic technologies required to perform remote surgeries so that they become used to the differences between in-person and remote procedures. One consideration is that there may be minute but noticeable delays in the technology, so they need to learn what these delays feel like and how to adjust for them. Although haptic feedback is currently being investigated for robotic surgery applications, there are still numerous issues to be resolved and very few haptic feedback options exist in current robotic systems. Thus, telesurgeons cannot rely on haptic feedback to guide their motions and reactions as they do with in-person procedures. They need to learn to rely more heavily on visual feedback and feedback from those actually present with the patient to gauge their actions and reactions.

One point regarding older surgeons and robotic/telesurgery applications should be made. In some respects the use of robotics may actually be of benefit to an older surgeon who still has all the necessary skills and expertise but is starting to suffer from subtle decreases in hand steadiness. Robotic systems essentially eliminate variations between surgeons in terms of hand steadiness and generally compensate for lack of steadiness. The use of robotics and telesurgery may actually extend the careers of some surgeons who otherwise would have had to stop or limit their practices.

4.6 Telerehabilitation

Telerehabilitation refers to the use of telehealth technologies for the delivery of rehabilitation services, including patient assessment (focusing on patients' functional abilities and their environment) and the delivery of therapeutic interventions. Telehealth tools and applications in this context are designed for several domains, including speech-language pathology, audiology, occupational and physical therapy, and neuropsychology. The types of telerehabilitation interventions that can be delivered are broad and include applications such as direct patient service delivery, specialist consultation, remote monitoring, and home telehealth and telerobotics (Brennan & Barker, 2008).

4.6.1 Factors to Consider in Telerehabilitation Consults

Human factors considerations can maximize the potential of telerehabilitation systems. While age, education, and technology experience of all involved users must be addressed when designing and implementing telehealth applications in general, in the context of telerehabilitation special consideration must be given to patients' potential impairments. Deficits in cognitive, gross or fine motor, visual, language, or voice skills play a significant role in patients' abilities to use software or hardware systems and accept their use in the context of health care. Telehealth technology for rehabilitation should be designed to provide features that maximize a patient's abilities while reducing the implications resulting from lost or impaired abilities. Established universal design principles can facilitate this goal. Examples include multiple modalities for human–computer interaction (e.g., including keyboards, touch screens and voice recognition as available platforms for data entry); accessible features such as large button telephones, simplified text-based interfaces; available resources for assistance (e.g., built-in troubleshooting features in addition to instruction manuals using text or graphic format); and considerations for the placement of hardware within a setting to address optimal environmental conditions (including light, space, minimizing interference with other daily activities).

4.6.2 Environmental Factors

More specifically, the environmental conditions need to be considered. The design of telerehabilitation space, whether it is within an institutional or residential setting, should enable patients with mobility aids such as walkers and wheelchairs to fully access the system if they are meant to be end-users, and minimize cluttering or other distractions. For traumatic brain injury patients with decreased levels of attention, it is important to design system interfaces that enable users to achieve tasks with few steps and no distractions. For patients with impaired speech or language, the audio and video quality of videoconferencing solutions needs to be tested extensively to ensure that technical quality challenges do not impede communication further between clinicians and patients. These examples highlight the need to fully understand the profile of potential end users and document their abilities, needs, and expectations. Furthermore, systems need to provide flexibility and account for changes in abilities and needs of patients over time. Finally, alternative educational techniques and informed consent procedures ensure all participants are able to fully understand the system procedures and tasks that will be required of them.

4.6.3 Some Interesting Applications

In the context of telerehabilitation there is the need for visual feedback, where in many instances motion and details of posture and gait need to be visually captured and thus requiring high-quality video signal transmission. Telerehabilitation applications have importance especially for rural settings where rehabilitation services are often lacking. Rural older patients discharged from rehabilitation hospitals face formidable barriers on return to the community. Access to health care in general and rehabilitation services in particular is more difficult for rural residents. Distance to facilities, transportation problems, rural poverty, and lack of rural service providers pose serious service access barriers for rural residents with disabilities. Lack of access to specialty services and new technologies prevent rural residents with disabilities from receiving appropriate services. Rural residents reported more chronic health problems and poorer general health, and perceived themselves as being less healthy than urban residents. Rural residents using home health services had higher levels of overall impairments in daily activities and poorer prognosis than comparable urban residents (Adams et al., 2001). These data highlight the elevated risk for exacerbation of chronic problems and secondary conditions for rural patients. The further rehabilitation programs are from rural residents' homes, the less likely they are to receive services.

While rural populations may be in greater need of telerehabilitation services, they may in many instances have less sophisticated infrastructure to support the implementation of telehealth solutions. Several projects have demonstrated that low-cost solutions in telerehabilitation have the potential to deliver effective services, including, for example, the use of a low-bandwidth, Internet-based telerehabilitation system to provide outpatient rehabilitation to patients who have undergone total knee arthroplasty. Telemedicine can enable a physical therapist from a metropolitan rehabilitation center to provide neurodevelopmental treatment to a patient in a nursing home, or support families providing in-home care for family members with prolonged states of reduced consciousness. There are Web-based telerehabilitation systems for arm and hand therapy following stroke that consist of a Web-based library of status tests, therapy games, and progress charts. The systems can be used with a variety of input devices, such as a low-cost force-feedback joystick, capable of assisting or resisting in movement. Data from home-based device usage by chronic stroke survivors demonstrates the feasibility of using the system for several purposes, including direction of therapy to mechanically assist in movement and to track improvements in movement ability.

4.6.4 Telehaptics

Recent advances in telehaptics are accelerating the growth of telerehabilitation. Telehaptics refers to the transmission of computer-generated tactile sensations to create a "sense" of touch. Such transmission is based on the use of sensors (including temperature, pressure, kinesthetic sensing, and biofeedback systems) and effectors (that create human sensations as outputs). Telehaptic interactivity provides sensed inputs such as brain activity, heartbeats, or breathing in an output format that triggers bodily sensations (such as warmth, pressure, vibration). This platform introduces new options for communication and a new dimension for interpersonal interaction during a telehealth encounter. Existing telerehabilitation system interfaces are already used to sample position of body parts (e.g., hands, elbows, knees) and provide resistive forces (e.g., using a virtual reality glove).

4.7 Telemental Health

Remote provision of support to mentally and emotionally distressed people began in earnest with the development of telephone networks (such as the 999 emergency number in the UK in the 1930s) and continues to this day with counseling services in many American cities using specialized crisis hotlines (e.g., 911, 211). For the most part, telemental health involves remote delivery of mental health services. The most important components are diagnosis and treatment, as well as continuing education for professionals. As in other fields of telemedicine, ensuring privacy and confidentiality of health communications and data is an important feature, but particularly in the case of mental health records, given the stigma still associated with mental health disorders. Here we will be concerned with factors that could affect diagnostic accuracy as well as treatment effectiveness.

4.7.1 Diagnostic Accuracy

Many consultations involve the use of videoconferencing equipment, with a therapist on one end and a client on the other. However, remote administration of diagnostic questionnaires such as standardized depression scales can also be accomplished through store-and-forward techniques, including postal mail (when delays are acceptable) and through dedicated small screen devices that can be attached to phone lines. The latest trend is to administer such instruments via smartphones, though the small screens in use at the present time may make text difficult to perceive by those older adults with presbyopia and particularly by those with more severe visual impairments (e.g., cataracts, glaucoma, age-related macular degeneration). Greater use of speech for input and output with such devices may help.

It is possible to use speech generation and recognition technologies to automate questionnaire administration over phones, though this procedure may create comprehension and memory difficulties for older adults (e.g., in remembering alternatives). Videoconference systems continue to improve in terms of visual image and sound quality due to better compression schemes for encoding and decoding information, coupled with higher bandwidth available for transmission of information. Nonetheless, particularly for packet-based transmission systems (e.g., using Internet transmission protocols that do not involve dedicated connections from end to end), quality can suffer during an extended session.

Degraded visual and auditory connections can potentially interfere with diagnostic testing. As an example, a popular screening device for assessing dementia contains immediate and delayed memory tests using a short list of spoken words. If the words spoken by the clinician are degraded in transmission, it may be difficult to determine if the problem experienced by the client for correctly repeating the words is due to memory impairment or to perceptual impairment. For instance, with age there is greater susceptibility to masking of signals by noise, which might occur for a degraded auditory channel. If the visual information is degraded, then older adults who rely on visual cues to interpret speech (lip reading) may be less able to compensate for auditory degradation.

Additional research is needed to determine whether remote testing and in-person testing yield the same or similar scores, though the few published studies suggest that scores obtained in teleconference conditions are highly correlated with those obtained with traditional in-person administration. Adopting a somewhat more lenient scoring criterion for determining accuracy in answering questions may be one practical approach to administering cognitive tests remotely. The research literature has shown that diagnostic assessment (e.g., score obtained on a rating scale) is comparable in videoconferencing and in-person evaluations, though there are relatively few high-quality investigations and these often use small sample sizes so are insensitive to small differences that may be clinically significant. One meta-analysis found that bandwidth of equipment was a moderator variable, in that higher quality videoconferencing minimized differences. That study did not investigate other than direct channels (dedicated lines).

Given the increased availability of low-cost computers, broadband, high definition webcams, and free videoconferencing software in homes, it is not unrealistic to imagine that a high percentage of households will soon be reachable for telemental health provision using the Internet. However, ensuring secure transmissions over the Internet is still problematic and hence may not meet professional and legal standards (for instance, Health Insurance Portability and Accountability Act (HIPAA) standards in the United States).

4.7.2 Treatment Effectiveness

Talk therapy is an important component of telemental health care provision. Establishing rapport with a client is usually a prerequisite for effective therapy. Thus the primary risk to the therapeutic relationship with distance care is degradation in the quality of the interaction between the professional and the client. As described above for other telemedicine specialties, trying to ensure that there is clarity in visual and auditory channels is important. Avoiding distracting features (e.g., the therapist wearing striped clothing, which often produces distracting visual artifacts with video transmission) may be particularly important for those with the least experience with this form of technology, namely older adults. Maintaining the appearance of direct eye contact is also more difficult to accomplish with videoconferencing, although in some cultures direct gaze may not be appreciated.

Given how difficult it is to find effects of therapist experience on therapeutic outcome (e.g., outcome differences between novices and experienced clinicians have been shown to be minimal), artifacts in videoconferencing sessions may have relatively little impact on therapeutic effectiveness. To this point there are few studies available to assess differences between in-person and videoconferencing therapy on outcomes aside from patient satisfaction measures.

Access to mental health care professionals is sorely lacking in rural communities where seniors tend to live, as well as in institutional settings such as nursing homes and prisons (sentencing practices in the United States have led to aging prison populations). Providing care via telemental health is one potentially important way to fill these gaps and to do so in a cost effective way by minimizing travel time.

4.8 Home Telehealth and Remote Monitoring

Telehealth in home care relies on the use of information technologies to enable health care providers at the clinical site to communicate with patients at their home. Telehealth can also enable patients to capture information about their well-being and become involved in their own care management.

Several telehealth applications in home care also use a videoconferencing component, allowing patients to see and hear a health care provider. Such an interaction via videoconferencing is often referred to as a "virtual visit" to distinguish it from actual face-to-face home health visits.

4.8.1 Mobile Health Applications

With the advancement of mobile health applications and the diffusion of the Internet, several telehealth applications for home care have emerged. Commercially available portable medical devices can easily be integrated into monitoring units, including portable spirometers, pulse oximeters, portable ECGs, and blood pressure devices. In some cases a more advanced application of patient monitoring can be implemented through wearable sensors. Most commercially available home telehealth units include a series of peripheral devices to capture vital signs, an interface that allows users to answer daily standardized questions, and in many cases a videophone feature to allow for virtual visits.

Human factors considerations should aim to reduce or minimize the "obtrusiveness" of telehealth. The home setting calls for this emphasis because the home is defined as a person's private and personal space; thus introduction of technology has a different psychological dynamic in the home environment than in an institutional facility. Obtrusiveness in home telehealth technology is defined as a summary evaluation by the user based on characteristics or effects associated with the technology that is perceived as undesirable and physically or psychologically prominent.

4.8.2 Installing Devices in Patients' Homes

Considerations pertaining to installation include the importance of system features that are physically integrated into the architecture and space and that do not clash with users' aesthetic sensibilities. The system specifications must address the existing residential infrastructure and a potential need for retrofitting. For example, several telehealth systems require high-speed Internet for data transmission or "virtual visits" to take place. Other systems rely on regular wired phone service with POTS (plain old telephone service), which may not be available as consumers often opt to eliminate landlines. Whether the existing infrastructure meets the system requirements and whether a potential upgrade or modification is possible should be the first set of considerations.

The actual residential conditions also need to be investigated. In many cases, cluttered space leaves little room for monitoring stations and peripheral devices to be safely installed. Additional considerations include the lighting of the room, which may affect the picture quality on a video screen or the visibility of data displays for monitoring devices; the potential hazard introduced by cables or other hardware components that may interfere with daily activities; and aesthetic concerns that residents may have with the placement of monitoring stations in areas visible to visitors.

4.8.3 Device Operation Considerations

Once the telehealth system is installed, its actual operation involves significant human factor considerations. Monitoring devices are in many cases tested with younger users even though their largest segment of the actual target population is older adults. Therefore, the interfaces of portable spirometers or blood pressure devices or even digital weight scales are not always appropriate for older adults with hearing or visual impairment. Research and evaluation projects of telehealth in home care indicate that older adults frequently relied on a family member or caregiver to operate or assist in the operation of devices and other hardware. Family caregivers in many cases fear that this will mean that a greater burden for providing care is placed on them. Furthermore, such a reliance on other stakeholders to assume the training and operation of telehealth equipment limits the potential users of home telehealth, as many older adults who are diagnosed with chronic conditions and aim to retain their independence live alone.

The usability of home telehealth units is critical. Older adults in home care or disease management programs may have functional limitations due to aging or their clinical diagnoses. A functional limitation describes a reduced sensory, cognitive, or motor capability that prevents a person from maximally functioning in an environment where others can. While it is often argued that advanced technologies have the potential to empower patients, older adults, who are the fastest growing segment of the U.S. population, are at a disadvantage, as system designers often fail to consider them as a target user group. Web interfaces are a critical component of several of the home telehealth applications. The design of a usable web information system for healthy users with extensive computer experience is a challenge. When a system needs to address age-related constraints and the functional limitations of potentially inexperienced users, the design challenge increases. Designers of a system for older adult home care patients should aim to increase its functional accessibility and ensure that actual users are involved in all phases of design and implementation.

If the telehealth system is to be operated by older adults, there is a need for training and an operations manual and other material that can help them deal with the regular planned operating steps as well as problem-solve unexpected difficulties. When developing training materials, it is important to maximize clarity and readability of the documentation. The use of examples, pictures, and detailed instructions can assist users who have never operated similar software or hardware devices before. It is often important to provide explanation for terms that may be very familiar to people with extensive computer usage experience (such as "drag and drop," "highlight," etc.) but may be foreign to those who have not used computers before. In addition to detailed manuals, users can benefit from quick overview visual summaries that they can choose to keep next to the telehealth station to remind themselves of regular steps and shortcuts.

4.8.4 Privacy and Security

A significant dimension of obtrusiveness is the concern for privacy loss. This pertains to both informational and physical privacy within the home setting. Informational privacy refers to the desire to control the sharing of personal information and may be violated when telehealth devices reveal more information than the user desires or raise this concern among users, whether it is a substantiated concern or not. Similarly, physical privacy is related to both the degree to which one is physically accessible to others and the accessibility of one's personal space or territory and may be a concern when telehealth technology is perceived to or actually impinges on the user's control of such access. In many cases, when videophone technology is used in the home, even if both parties have to consent to conduct a video call, it helps address privacy concerns for users when the camera is covered to ensure that no third party would be able to remotely turn the camera on. Furthermore, a clear explanation of the data transmission procedures and the safety of the actual data repositories as well as a discussion of all parties who have access to the data help address privacy concerns. The challenge is to provide explanations that allow people to understand the procedures even if they have no experience or knowledge of data transmission logistics or Internet protocols. Ensuring that the system is in a physical location that also satisfies privacy expectations further addresses this concern.

4.8.5 Maintenance of Home Health Devices

Finally, human factors issues inform considerations addressing the maintenance of the telehealth system in the home. Many portable devices need regular change of batteries. Additionally, spirometry and glucose meter devices call for specific cleaning and maintenance procedures. A system needs to be in place to remind users of maintenance needs of the hardware components and to ensure that such procedures can be carried out by the older adult user or provisions are made for a health care provider or other third party to carry these out. It is essential that the actual use of telehealth in the home is observed or at least evaluated based on the residents' self-report. The use of telehealth technology in the home may affect users' daily routines or rituals or require the acquisition of new ones. The home care literature highlights how introducing durable medical equipment, such as hospital beds, Hoyer lifts, and bedside commodes, can affect personal routines within the home. It is important to manifest whether telehealth technology brought into the home can also be perceived as obtrusive to personal routines and activities of daily living in the same way.

4.8.6 Personal Health Records

In recent years the concept of personal health records has gained increased attention as a potential approach to owning and managing one's own health data. Emerging from the proliferation of Internet access in individual residences, the term personal health record (PHR) has now become the term that describes the electronic record of one's health-related data, or as the National Alliance for Health Information Technology defines it, "an individual's electronic record of health-related information that conforms to nationally recognized interoperability standards and that can be drawn from multiple sources while being managed, shared and controlled by the individual."

A PHR is meant to be a tool that empowers individuals by enabling them to share health information, increase access to educational resources, and engage multiple stakeholders in the health care process. For this reason, PHR applications are envisioned as a platform that shifts from institution-centric to patient-centric models of care. The individual patient or consumer in general becomes the owner and manager of his or her health data. PHR systems featured by Google (Google Health) and Microsoft (HealthVault) are conceptualized along these premises to provide consumers with access to their own health information without specific hardware requirements or organizational agreements.

PHR systems hold great potential in the context of home based telehealth monitoring and can therefore play a role in the care of older adults, supporting disease prevention and management as well as wellness promotion. While PHR use specifically for older adults has not yet been extensively examined, several research studies have highlighted the challenges that elders face or may face when using PHR systems. Such challenges may include computer literacy, the digital divide, and access to appropriate software and hardware resources to ensure successful adoption of PHR systems among older adults. One study explored the use and utility of PHRs in a low-income, elderly population (Kim, et al., 2009). The three-year study involved 44 elderly residents of a federally funded housing facility. Researchers assessed use and user satisfaction of a Web-based PHR called the Personal Health Information Management System (PHIMS). Use among the residents was low, with only 13% of eligible residents using the system, and of those about half only used the system on one day. This study concluded that the majority of the low-income elderly would not be in a position to benefit from PHRs due to poor technical skills, technophobia, low health literacy, and limited physical/cognitive abilities.

The proliferation rates of Internet usage among older adults obviously affect adoption rates for PHR systems. A large, systematic survey of US veterans' Internet use confirmed prior findings that age was correlated negatively with greater Internet use (McInnes et al., 2010). However, one interesting result in terms of the older adults was that among Internet-using veterans, there was no effect of age on health-related Internet use. Fonda et al. also examined older adults' needs in a study that reported on the creation of a prototype for a personal health application (PHA) for patients with both type 1 and type 2 diabetes (Fonda et al., 2010). Participants emphasized their preference for a personal health tool that provides accurate, timely, readily available information on how diabetes-related domains interact, how their own behaviors affect diabetes, and what to do next when faced with new information.

Once personal health-related information is stored in one online repository, the challenge becomes how to display the data sets in a meaningful way and how to highlight trajectories over time. Capturing overarching concepts important to older adults, such as wellness or quality of life, requires the use of visualization tools that will most efficiently capture information both on a macro level (assessing the overall pattern or status) and on a micro level (examining trends for individual parameters over time). Curran (1999) has argued that one way to reduce the cognitive effort required to understand quantitative information is to present the data in a graphical display, especially when the data are intended to showcase changes over time. In this context, various theories of graphical comprehension can be applied. Shaw's cognitive model for understanding information (Shaw et al., 1999) displayed graphically includes three phases: a search for visual qualitative information; a search for quantitative relationships; and a subsequent integration of both that allows the reader to interpret the graph. A graph allows the user to process quantitative information in a format that is easier to understand and retain than a textual presentation. Considerations for the design of graphic interfaces for older adults can inform the design of visualization approaches in the context of PHR systems as well in order to maximize comprehension and utility of personal health information.

4.9 Summary

Some common themes emerge from the review of telemedicine specialties. Most disciplines rely on real-time videoconferencing or store-and-forward technologies to diagnose and treat clients. One of the threats to effectiveness is the reliance on less-well-trained staff at remote locations to collect and transmit the high quality data that the specialist desires. Another threat is that store-and-forward technologies can introduce significant delays in transmission of information that can jeopardize health in time-critical situations. Older adults who are less familiar with technology than their younger counterparts may have significant concerns about telemedicine that require reassurance. Older health care professionals and their clients typically experience degraded perceptual, cognitive, and motor capabilities that can be further hampered by losses in quality during transmission of information to and from remote locations.

Many of these concerns can be met be designing better technology (e.g., videoconferencing systems) that take human capabilities into account, particularly age-related changes in abilities. Others can be met by better education and training for users. Given the difficulties in transporting specialist care to remote locations, telehealth technologies offer a potentially cost effective way to support those in need.

4.10 Suggested Readings

Adams, C., Michel, Y., DeFrates, D., and Corbett, C. (2001). Effect of locale on health status and direct care time of rural versus urban home health patients. *Journal of Nursing Administration*, 31, 244–51.

Brennan, D.M., and Barker, L.M. (2008). Human factors in the development and implementation of telerehabilitation systems. *Journal of Telemedicine and Telecare*, 14, 55–58.

Curran, C.R. (1999). Data display techniques. *Applied Nursing Research*, 12(3), 153–58.

Fonda, S.J., Kedziora, R.J., Vigersky, R.A., and Bursell, S.E. (2010). Combining iGoogle and personal health records to create a prototype personal health application for diabetes self-management. *Telemedicine Journal and E-Health*, 16(4), 480–89.

Hensel, B.K., Demiris, G., and Courtney, K.L. (2006). Defining obtrusiveness in home telehealth technologies: A conceptual framework. *Journal of the American Medical Informatics Association*, 13(4), 428–31.

Hyler, S.E., Gangure, D.P., and Batchelder, S.T. (2005). Can telepsychiatry replace in-person psychiatric assessments? A review and meta-analysis of comparison studies. *CNS Spectrums*, 10, 403–13.

Kim, E.H., Stolyar, A., Lober, W.B., Herbaugh, A.L., Shinstrom, S.E., Zierler, B.K., Soh, C.B., and Kim, Y. (2009). Challenges to using an electronic personal health record by a low-income elderly population. *Journal of Medical Internet Research,* 11(4):e44. Retrieved from http://www.jmir.org/2009/4/e44/.

McInnes, D.K., Gifford, A.L., Kazis, L.E., and Wagner, T.H. (2010). Disparities in health-related internet use by US veterans: Results from a national survey. *Informatics in Primary Care,* 18(1), 59–68.

Pickering, G., Jourdan, D., Eschalier, A., and Dubray, C. (2002). Impact of age, gender and cognitive functioning on pain perception. *Gerontology,* 48:112–18. DOI: 10.1159/000048937.

Rabinowitz, T., Brennan, D.M., Chumbler, N.R., Kobb, R., and Yellowlees, P. (2008). New directions for telemental health research. *Telemedicine and e-Health,* 14, 972–76.

Reinkensmeyer, D.J., Pang, C.T., Nessler, J.A., and Painter, C.C. (2002). Web-based telerehabilitation for the upper extremity after stroke. *IEEE Transactions on Neural Systems and Rehabilitation Engineering,* 10(2), 102–8.

Shaw, P.A., Mayer, R.E., and Hagarty, M. (1999). Graphs as aids to knowledge construction: Signaling techniques for guiding the process of graph comprehension. *Journal of Educational Psychology,* 91, 690–72.

chapter 5

Standards and Guidelines

In this chapter we highlight telehealth-related associations and the guidelines that they have developed for telehealth systems.

5.1 The American Telemedicine Association and Standards

The American Telemedicine Association (ATA) was established in 1993 as a nonprofit organization to bring together groups from such areas as medicine, academia, technology, telecommunications, and government to overcome barriers to the advancement of telemedicine (see www.americantelemed.org). The association works to achieve this goal through a variety of mission-related activities. One of its main activities is to create the basis for assuring uniform quality in the delivery of remote health care services, particularly via the Standards and Guidelines Committee efforts. There are also a number of professional societies associated with the numerous clinical specialties that use telemedicine that have created and endorsed standards, guidelines, and clinical practice recommendations.

Although none of these documents has addressed human factors specifically, they all do contain specific information regarding the best ways to use various pieces of equipment, how to best communicate with patients, and the environmental conditions that should be established (e.g., room design) for the best practice of telemedicine. Likewise, none of the documents deals specifically with older patients, but again the best practice recommendations have been well thought out for general patient populations and can be interpreted and adapted for use with older patient populations.

Telemedicine is a broad field that includes nearly every clinical subspecialty being practiced today. It is therefore impractical, and likely not necessary, to develop standards and guidelines for every possible clinical specialty or telemedicine application. Recognizing this, the ATA decided to focus initially on a core set of principles that would guide telemedicine practice in general. The initial effort created a Telemedicine/Telehealth Glossary of Terms composed of terms and definitions commonly used in telemedicine/telehealth. It was assembled to encourage consistency in employing these terms throughout the telemedicine enterprise.

5.1.1 Core Standards for Telemedicine Operations

The Core Standards for Telemedicine Operations document was completed in 2007 (ATA, 2007), and covers broad policies and procedures that should be used by institutions providing remote medical services, interactive patient encounters, and any other electronic communications between patients and practitioners for the purposes of health care delivery. It includes the idea that the standards apply to individual practitioners, group practices, health care systems, and other providers of health-related services where there are telehealth interactions between patients and service providers for the purposes of health care delivery. It provides guidance with respect to the administrative, clinical, and technical aspects of telemedicine practice.

5.1.2 Administrative Standards

The Administrative Standards section deals with issues of responsibility and standard operating procedures. Briefly, it states that organizations and providers shall follow standard operating policies and procedures of the governing institution, especially with respect to human resource management; privacy and confidentiality; federal, state, and other credentialing and regulatory agency requirements; fiscal management; ownership of patient records; documentation; patient rights and responsibilities; network security; telehealth equipment use; and research protocols.

Quality improvement and assessment procedures shall be in place, as are all other aspects of patient care that require adherence to federal, state, and local regulatory bodies (i.e., patient consent, protection of health information, patient rights and responsibilities, integration of telemedicine into a practice, collaborative agreements/contracts). Health care professionals shall be fully licensed and registered, aware of credentialing requirements, aware of their locus of accountability, cognizant of when a provider–patient telehealth relationship has been established, and shall have the necessary education and training to ensure safe provision of health services. These administrative guidelines clearly do not differ from standard operating procedures that organizations and health professionals follow without involving telemedicine. They are designed to reiterate and emphasize that telemedicine needs to be carried out with the same high standards of patient care and safety that are normally followed.

5.1.3 Telemedicine Ethics

The section on telemedicine practice ethics states that although telemedicine is not a practice in and of itself, practicing at a distance does create a unique relationship with the patient that requires attention to and adherence to professional ethical principles that may be new to practitioners. The ethics section states that an organization or health care professional shall (1) incorporate organizational values and ethics statements into the administrative policies and procedures for telemedicine; (2) be aware of medical and other professional discipline codes of ethics when using telemedicine; and (3) inform patients of their rights and responsibilities when receiving care at a distance (through telemedicine), including to influence decisions made about, for, or with patients who receive care via telemedicine.

5.1.4 Clinical Guidelines and Standards

The Clinical Standards section acknowledges that practice guidelines will be different to some degree for every clinical specialty and are thus more fully dealt with in dedicated specialty guidelines. Only two major points are noted: (1) the organization and health professional shall be satisfied that health professionals providing care via telehealth are aware of their professional discipline standards and that those standards shall be upheld in telemedicine; and (2) health professionals shall be guided by existing professional discipline and national practice guidelines when practicing telehealth, and, if modifications exist specifically for telehealth, they shall be followed.

5.1.5 Technical Standards

The Technical Standards section deals with broad equipment and technology issues. It again notes that certain specialties will utilize equipment unique to their specialty, and thus more specific technical standards are provided in each specialty set of practice guidelines. The section does not deal specifically with human factors or different patient populations, but highlights the importance of such considerations. The technical standards include such aspects as ensuring the equipment used is available and properly functioning; that it meets all relevant laws, regulations and codes for safety; that infection control policies and procedures are in place; patient information is safe and complies with local and federal legislation and rules regarding privacy and confidentiality; that systems have appropriate redundancies in place, especially for network connectivity; that published technical standards are met for safety and efficacy of devices used with patients; and that equipment is properly maintained.

Although none of the documents deal explicitly with human factors issues, as noted they do so implicitly in many cases. For example, the Telemental Health Videoconferencing guidelines (ATA, 2009) discuss cultural competency and the need for the teleclinician to understand cultural differences and how they may influence the patient–clinician interaction.

This guideline also addresses older patients, noting that they often have sensory deficits that can impair their ability to interact over a videoconferencing system so the type of technology used should be considered carefully. They also note that with older patients family members should be included as appropriate, and interview techniques should be adjusted for patients who may be cognitively impaired.

5.2 ATA Guidelines

To date, the ATA has created the following standards and guidelines documents that are all freely available on the ATA website (www.americantelemed.org).

1. Core Standards for Telemedicine Operations
2. Practice Guidelines for Videoconferencing-Based Telemental Health
3. Evidence-Based Practice for Telemental Health
4. Practice Guidelines for Teledermatology
5. Telehealth Practice Recommendations for Diabetic Retinopathy
6. Home Telehealth Clinical Guidelines
7. Clinical Guidelines for Telepathology

Other clinical specialties such as teleradiology have created their own sets of guidelines specific to their clinical subspecialty (Seibert et al., 2004; VanMoore et al., 2005).

Developing guidelines and standards for telemedicine is an important and valuable process for ensuring effective and safe delivery of quality health care. The practice guidelines developed to date have been well-received by the telemedicine community and are being adopted in numerous practices. As telemedicine grows and is adopted by more health care practitioners in their regular clinical practice, more practice guidelines will be created and adopted. As more patient populations are exposed to telemedicine, it seems likely that these guidelines will start to incorporate more explicit references to geriatric and other unique populations.

5.3 National and International Standards and Guidelines

There are still relatively few national and international standards for telehealth. One national (US) source of information specific to human factors considerations for medical devices is ANSI/AAMI HE-75 (http://www.aami.org/publications/standards/he75.html). The International Organization for Standards (ISO) has several documents that can be consulted for telehealth, such as for health informatics (ISO 21667:2010). There also are standards concerning specific devices such as glucose meters (ISO/IEEE 11073-10417:2010), blood pressure monitors (ISO/IEEE 11073-10407:2010), and pulse oximeters (ISO/IEEE 11073-10404:2010). These can be found on its website: http://www.iso.org/iso/home.htm. Also relevant is a set of guidelines for addressing the needs of older people and people with disabilities (http://www.iso.org/iso/catalogue_detail?csnumber=40933).

5.4 Suggested Readings

American Telemedicine Association Standards and Guidelines. (2010). Retrieved from http://www.americantelemed.org/i4a/pages/index.cfm?pageID=3311.

American Telemedicine Association's Core Standards for Telemedicine Operations. (2007). Retrieved from http://www.americantelemed.org/files/public/standards/CoreStandards_withCOVER.pdf.

American Telemedicine Association's Practice Guidelines for Videoconferencing-Based Telemental Health. Retrieved from http://www.americantelemed.org/i4a/pages/index.cfm?pageID=3311.

Seibert, J.A., Kent, J.S., & Geiss, R.A. (2004). Practice guideline for electronic medical information privacy and security. Retrieved from http://www.acr.org/SecondaryMainMenuCategories/quality_safety/guidelines/med_phys/electronic_medical_info.aspx.

Van Moore, A., Allen, B., & Campbell, S.C. (2005). Report of the ACR task force on international teleradiology. *Journal of the American College of Radiology*, 2, 121–5.

chapter 6

Tutorials on Usability Testing, Setting up Diagnostics, and Health Status Monitoring

Our aim in this chapter is to provide the reader with practical tips on how to ensure that telehealth systems work as planned. The process should involve both usability testing and tips and guidelines for deploying the systems. We begin with a discussion of usability testing, then discuss setting up diagnostics, and end with a brief discussion of the issues in detecting critical health conditions and the problem of false alarms.

6.1 Usability Testing

Given variability in the environment, almost all telehealth equipment installations will require some adjustments. Similarly, given variability in the capabilities of users, almost all telehealth interventions will require user training for both the health care practitioner and the client. Thus it will usually be necessary to test a system to assure that tasks can be carried out as intended. Usability testing is a collection of methodologies aimed at evaluating the extent of person–environment fit illustrated in Figure 1.1 (Chapter 1).

There are two broad and overlapping approaches to usability testing: (1) problem discovery and (2) performance assessment. The former is usually concerned with uncovering difficulties and hence focuses on user error (and redesign to remediate flaws), and the latter is concerned with promoting efficient achievement of goals and hence focuses on time to complete a unit task with the system (e.g., complete a surgical procedure using telesurgery equipment). Usability testing can be employed with both developing systems (during the design process) and with mature systems to assess performance in a range of environments (e.g., a traditional hospital setting versus a telemedicine clinic or a home).

Sample size: An important issue to consider for usability testing is how many participants to enroll for a test, and this becomes even more critical when specialized users (e.g., health care professionals) are part of the testing panel. The two (conflicting) factors here are cost and power. Cost refers to the expense of conducting the research. Participants may need to be reimbursed for the time that they commit to a test session or sessions. There is also a cost associated with collecting and analyzing the data. Another cost factor is the cost of failing to find significant design problems or flaws, particularly those that might threaten the safety of the user of the telehealth system. Correcting undetected problems that appear only after deployment can be quite expensive.

Power refers to the likelihood of finding significant design flaws. One can think of this issue as similar to the problem of obtaining a winning ticket from a raffle at a fundraising event. Some raffles have multiple winning tickets (design flaws) and others have just one. Some raffles might sell 1,000 tickets before the draw is made (hence creating a low probability of obtaining a winning ticket or design flaw for those buying only a few tickets), and others might sell only 100, making it easier to win when buying a large block of tickets. Clearly buying more tickets—testing more participants—increases the chance of winning (finding a winning ticket or tickets, or here, a design flaw). By testing every possible user on all possible tasks it is possible to discover all the flaws. That approach is obviously impractical. But it remains true that the more people tested, the more flaws are typically uncovered, with diminishing returns as sample size increases beyond some optimal number. Flaws may have high or low probabilities of occurring in a particular test with a particular user. One favorable feature for usability testing with an older population is that older adults tend to be less robust for perceptual, cognitive, and psychomotor processing. Hence they uncover design flaws more readily than younger adults. Thus in general, smaller panels of older adults are needed to uncover flaws.

Assume that based on prior research, there is already an estimate of the probability of a flaw occurring. If so, there are tables that can be consulted to set sample size for usability testing. See Lewis (2006). Here we restrict consideration to the simplified case where a single occurrence of a flaw is reason to try to correct it, though one could also consider cases where it would be required to occur twice (or more often) before triggering a design correction. There are two parameters that need to be considered for setting an appropriate sample size: p, the probability of a flaw occurring in the usability test, and c, the confidence level that is appropriate to set for detecting flaws. The binomial distribution can be used to estimate the probability, p, of detecting a flaw at least once for a given sample size, n, using formula (1).

$$\text{Flaw detection} = 1 - (1 - p)^n \quad (1)$$

Figure 6.1 shows the curves as a function of different probabilities of occurrence for a flaw.

Take the example of a design flaw that has a probability of occurring of 0.01, the nearly straight line at the bottom of Figure 6.1. With a sample

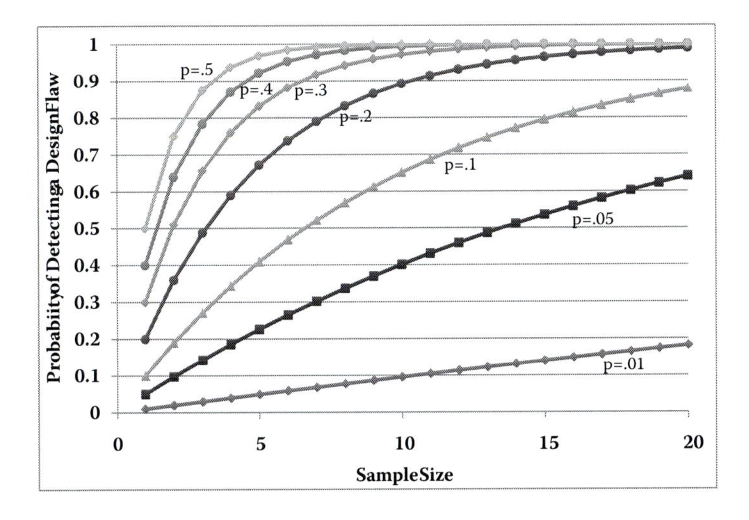

Figure 6.1 Probability of detecting a design flaw as a function of sample size for different probabilities of appearance of a design flaw, ranging from p = 0.01 in the lower right curve to p = 0.5 in the upper left curve.

size of 1 participant, the probability of it appearing is p = 0.01. With a sample size of 20, the probability of detecting that flaw rises to nearly p = 0.2. Chances are obviously much better for detection if the probability of the problem arising increases. So for the curve for a probability of 0.05 (a 1 in 20 chance of appearing), by doing usability testing with 20 participants there is nearly a 65% chance of observing that flaw. If the flaw is glaring, say for the case of the top curve, p = 0.5, then all it takes is 3 participants before usability testing is almost 90% likely to detect that problem.

The next step in deciding on sample size is to consider the appropriate criterion to set for detecting a flaw. That is, it is necessary to set a confidence level for detecting flaws. A common level for power analyses of sample size is to have a probability of p = 0.8 for detecting the flaw. So if flaws occur with moderate probabilities, say in the p = 0.1 to p = 0.4 range, then having between 3 and 15 participants will generally enable near 80% detection. However, if flaws might lead to safety problems, a higher probability should be set (confidence of 0.9 or 0.95). It is possible to derive a formula to encompass the two factors of the probability of the flaw arising during testing, p, and the confidence level, c, that the human factors specialist chooses. It is shown in formula 2, given in Lewis (2006).

$$\text{Sample size} = \log(1-c)/\log(1-p) \qquad (2)$$

As an example, suppose that a design flaw will be seen with p = 0.1 and that the investigator wants to be 90% confident (c = 0.9) of catching a design flaw. Substituting those values into the formula yields a projected sample size for testing of log (1-0.9)/log(1-0.1) or log (0.1)/log(0.9). Taking the logs yields a ratio of -1/-0.04576 = 21.8 participants. This can be rounded up to 22 participants. This result meshes with what is graphed in Figure 6.1, which ends with n = 20. The formula provides a simple method to calculate an appropriate sample size for usability testing.

As in the process of design itself, usability testing involves tradeoffs between costs and benefits. Larger usability samples consume more time and resources than smaller samples when testing telehealth systems but yield a higher probability of detecting flaws. As mentioned earlier, because older adults are more sensitive to design flaws, they make ideal participants in usability testing. Alan Welford, one of the pioneers of human factors and aging, noted many years ago that older participants will show you flaws in a product much more readily than younger adults. They make ideal critics.

When there is little prior research to establish the probability of occurrence of a flaw, a good strategy is to test a few individuals initially. Tally the flaws detected and calculate the probability of uncovering flaws, then increase the sample size to one that generates reasonable confidence in detecting currently undetected flaws using formula 2.

Usability testing may also involve more than problem discovery, as mentioned above. It also can involve performance assessment. Usability testing usually targets five major dimensions in evaluating performance with a telehealth system. The mnemonic "Let Every Mature Elder Succeed," LEMES, can help with remembering the relevant dimensions for evaluation: learnability, efficiency, memorability, errors, satisfaction.

Learnability refers to how easy it is to learn to use a system or tool. Learnability is usually assessed by giving the user the system, including training materials, and setting up tasks to be performed. How quickly can the naïve user learn what is necessary to perform the task? As an example, consider an older user who is unfamiliar with a videoconferencing system. How quickly can that user learn to initiate a videoconference session? One might set a goal of having the typical (average) user start a videoconferencing session within an hour of the time that a system is introduced into his or her home. Or one might put restrictions on the task, such as requiring that 90% of the new users must be able to carry out the task successfully without ever having to contact technical support staff. (Finding mean times to complete tasks should be preferred to finding percentages of a user group completing a task for statistical reasons involved in estimating percentiles of a population. Basically, a larger sample size is needed to estimate percentiles near the extremes of a distribution, usually sample sizes of 20 or more.) A typical laboratory test would be done in a controlled environment with a representative sampling of users if done during product development. A typical field test would involve a representative sampling of deployment environments (e.g., a home or apartment that a typical older adult might live in).

Efficiency refers to how quickly a user can accomplish a goal or objective of the system and takes into account factors such as fatigue or frustration while doing so. Some systems may be more efficient than others (take less time to accomplish the same goal, or take the same time but result in less fatigue or frustration). As an example, consider a comparison between two radiology display monitors that both show high resolution images at 1900 × 1200 pixels, but one provides a better light/dark contrast ratio, leading to lower eyestrain for extended use, and hence minimizes fatigue.

Memorability refers to how easily someone can return to using a system in an efficient way after a period of nonuse. Memorability is an important attribute for activities that are only performed occasionally (e.g., maintenance procedures for a medical device). Usually, if the system is easily learnable, it will also be easy to relearn. However, in the case of an older adult with clinical memory impairment, something that was easy to learn to use at an early stage of dementia might be very difficult to relearn to use at a moderate level of dementia. A test of memorability would entail the same process as testing learnability, but with the addition of a time interval. For example, is the mean time to carry out a task 60 seconds or fewer at one month after they were initially trained? For a percentage target, an example might be: can 90% of users still carry out a task successfully without recourse to technical support one month after they initially were trained to use the equipment or perform a procedure?

Errors in use are inevitable when working with any moderately complex system. Further, people, even when they are well-trained, also experience "slips," actions not as intended, when they accidentally press the wrong button on a control, particularly when they are under time pressure. So when designing a system or training people to use a system, it is extremely important to ensure that people are properly alerted to error states, can recover from errors when they occur, and that catastrophic (unrecoverable) errors are largely avoided. For instance, one might want to determine how robust a remote sensing system is (what state it returns to) following power spikes, brownouts, and complete power outages. It is necessary to test whether an older user will be seriously harmed if they accidentally repeat or omit a step in a multistep procedure when, for instance, using an oxygen concentrator at home.

The more steps in a procedure, the greater the likelihood of an error occurring at some point in the procedure. The exact form of this function, when errors are equally probable at each step, can be seen in Figure 6.2. Simply rename the *X*-axis to "number of steps in a procedure" and the *Y*-axis to "probability of an error occurring." The curves shown should be interpreted as the a priori probability of an error on a step. (The same binomial distribution function, formula 1, applies here.) In this case, for a

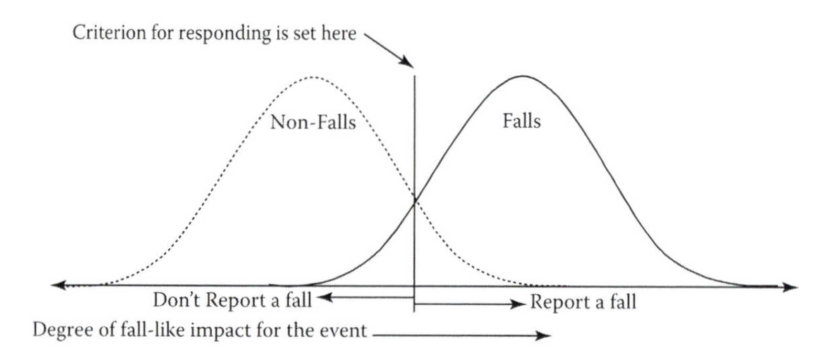

Figure 6.2 Nonfall and fall distributions overlapping on a "degree of impact" dimension and a criterion point for reporting the event as a fall.

person who is 95% reliable in carrying out any step—that is, has a p (error) = 0.05—there is about a 50% chance of making an error at some point in a 13-step procedure. Thus a good heuristic for design is to minimize the number of steps in a procedure.

Satisfaction testing assesses how satisfied users are with the operation of a system. Often simple questionnaires with rating scales can be used to assess satisfaction. However, one needs to be careful to assess different aspects of satisfaction. In general, the published literature shows that when people are given a new system to use at no cost, they are almost always very satisfied with it (gifts are usually positively rated). If possible one should assess how satisfaction changes over time given the high rate of abandonment (the drawer/closet problem) experienced for many consumer products, particularly assistive devices.

A useful collection of tools that can help with formal usability testing is provided at http://www.stcsig.org/usability/resources/toolkit/toolkit.html (accessed 11/7/10).

6.1.1 Recommendations

Sample size: For many usability testing situations, including between 5 and 15 participants should be adequate to detect many design flaws. When the cost of failing to find a flaw is high—for instance, when safety could be compromised—more participants should be tested.

6.2 Setting up Diagnostics

The key to setting up a diagnostic telemedicine program is planning. Diagnostic in this context refers to the conduct of patient–clinician consultations (or sometimes clinician–clinician consults), as opposed to simply administrative or educational sessions. Prior to actually purchasing any equipment, installing devices, or setting up clinics, it is necessary to carry out a site assessment. There is no single way to carry out such an assessment, but the National Library of Medicine has a very nice series of guides that can help.

Some of the key questions to ask in the initial assessment of a potential site to add to a telemedicine network are: what populations will be served, which communities are most in need, which communities can best be reached, what are the users of the service, what is needed and used, and what are the barriers? To help answer these questions, it is useful to access and review as many sources as possible. Use primary and secondary sources to analyze demographics, health status, and patterns of health care use. Talk to stakeholders—clinicians, chief executive officers, chief financial officers, chief information officers, and, perhaps most importantly, patient groups. A key goal is to determine if telemedicine will be accepted and used in a particular community before undertaking an endeavor that is not looked upon favorably from the start.

Once the site assessment has been completed, the equipment is being installed, and the clinicians brought on board, it is time to consider setting up diagnostics. The practice of telemedicine is becoming fairly well-established and used on a more regular basis by a wide variety of practices and clinical specialties. Although every environment and practice is unique to some extent, there are significant commonalities that should not be ignored. There is much that can be learned about how to set up a diagnostic telemedicine practice by reviewing the literature and going to scientific meetings. Even more beneficial is to attend one of the many training programs available at a variety of established telemedicine centers (e.g., the Arizona Telemedicine Program [http://www.telemedicine.arizona.edu/], the University of California Davis Telemedicine Program [http://www.ucdmc.ucdavis.edu/cht/services/telemedicine/]). Most of these programs hold one- or two-day courses that cover a broad range of topics, from basic technology through a variety of clinical subspecialties. The American Telemedicine Association also holds a variety of training courses for both the novice and intermediate telemedicine user at its annual meeting. If it is not possible to attend any of these options, try to find a telemedicine program in your area and schedule a visit to tour the program and talk with key personnel.

Another excellent resource is a group of federally funded telemedicine resource centers. In 2006 the Office for the Advancement of Telehealth (OAT) initiated a regional telehealth resource center grant program to provide support and guidance to telehealth programs. Currently there are five Telehealth Resource Centers (TRCs) and a Technology Assessment Center with the mission to serve as focal points for advancing the effective use of telehealth and support access to telehealth services in rural and underserved communities. More resource centers are expected to be funded in future years. Each TRC has extensive telehealth experience and can provide services, resources, and tools to telemedicine programs.

The key to setting up a successful and sustainable diagnostic telemedicine program is focus. Although some programs have had good success using a model that provides services in a wide variety of clinical subspecialties, the more commonly successful model is one that starts with one or a few basic services. The initial stage establishes these practices and then, if warranted and feasible, expands into other specialties. There are a few core clinical specialties that have been shown to readily serve as foundations upon which more services can be added. Teleradiology is probably one of the easiest telepractices to establish. The majority of radiology practice today is digitally based and has been for a number of years. Even small clinics utilize computed radiography and have some sort of Picture Archiving and Communications System on the premises. The addition of telecommunications capability is almost trivial in many environments, and clinics can easily and securely be connected to each other for teleradiology.

Acceptance of and satisfaction with teleradiology by both clinicians and patients has been high, perhaps because there is very little difference between teleradiology and traditional radiology. The majority of radiology (except interventional and a few other procedures) involves little to no contact between the radiologist and the patient. Images are acquired by a radiology technologist and transmitted to workstations in a reading room where the radiologist interprets them. The diagnostic report is generated (often electronically) and sent to the referring clinician and possibly the patient. The main difference in teleradiology is that the image acquisition site and the image interpretation site are not colocated and can be hundreds if not thousands of miles away from each other. Given the lack of significant differences between the practice of radiology and teleradiology, teleradiology is readily reimbursed and thus highly sustainable. The main lesson from radiology, with respect to setting up other diagnostic telemedicine practices, is to maintain as much of the traditional way of practicing as possible.

The hurdles for teleradiology were the same as those encountered when radiology went from a film-based practice to digital, and many of them centered around human factors issues. Initially, the acquisition technology had to be refined and optimized for digital acquisition of the radiographic images. For the most part, this was based in physics, chemistry, and electronics—developing detectors that had sufficient resolution (spatial and contrast), dynamic range, sensitivity, etc., to acquire images with at least as good quality as film. Today digital technology in radiology is solidly in place, and there are standards in place regarding image acquisition quality (Williams et al., 2007).

Other specialties are following the lead of teleradiology and are establishing standards and guidelines for the acquisition of images to be used in teleconsults. For example, the practice guidelines for teledermatology contain specific recommendations for camera resolution, white balance, metadata labeling, compression, and color bit-depth (Krupinski et al., 2007). The telemental health guidelines provide real-time videoconferencing specifications, including minimum bandwidth, transmission speed, and resolution and interoperability requirements (Grady et al., 2009). Many clinical specialties require the use of peripheral devices other than just cameras. Electronic stethoscopes, EKG/EMG/EEG devices, portable ultrasound, blood pressure monitors, spirometers, and so on are all being used in diagnostic telemedicine applications. Nearly all of them have been evaluated and used in some clinical situation, so there are data available in the literature, on websites, and by contacting those who have used them. Prior to selecting a device, it is important to get as much information as possible about its capabilities and limitations before purchasing it.

The human factors side of the equation in teleradiology came into play after the acquisition technology was established and the digital images needed to be displayed in a digital medium. As with acquisition, guidelines exist with respect to minimum recommended standards for the display of radiographic digital images (Krupinski et al., 2007). In any diagnostic telemedicine application, the overall goal in choosing the display device is to match the output of an imaging system to the display and then to optimize the display to the observer's visual system in a given reading environment. The former requires that the workstation match the spatial and dynamic resolution of the imaging system. For telemammography, medical grade monochrome displays are available with up to 5 M-pixels resolution and thus satisfy the spatial requirement for nearly every imaging modality. Teleradiology probably represents the extreme case for spatial resolution. Almost every other telemedicine application uses commercial off-the-shelf color displays, and as long as the display closely matches the resolution of the acquired image (or can zoom to it), the resolution is likely sufficient for the user to detect and discriminate the relevant diagnostic details.

Most telemedicine display guidelines take into account the human visual system capabilities. Recommended values for such key display parameters as minimum and maximum luminance, contrast ratio, matrix size, display size, bit depth, spatial resolution, pixel size, noise, veiling glare, and reflections can be found in the various standards documents.

One of the keys to a successful softcopy presentation of telemedicine images (mostly store and forward in this context, but many of the issues apply to real time as well) is the design of the workstation-user interface. It is the backbone of the telemedicine workstation, and optimizing it covers a wide range of issues, from technical and clinical to machine and human factors. It is affected by both hardware and software aspects. User interfaces should be fast, intuitive, user friendly, able to integrate and expand,

and reliable. In telemedicine there are a number of companies developing complete workstation solutions as well as dedicated software options for diagnostic telemedicine.

When selecting from these numerous options, the following should be considered. The user (e.g., clinician, site coordinator, other health care provider) should be able to use the basic navigation tools without extensive training and without prior exposure. The system should be user friendly and easy to customize. This includes simple menus and file managers, single mouse click navigation, visually comfortable colors, and an uncluttered workspace.

The type of input device used with a telemedicine workstation is often a matter of personal preference but should be chosen to be comfortable, especially over long periods of time, to avoid repetitive strain injuries such as carpal tunnel syndrome. Some of the most common choices include keyboards (preferably with hot key options to reduce the number of steps required to complete a procedure), mouse (with or without a scroll wheel and with various number and types of buttons), and track balls. The key to selecting an input device relates to user comfort and task. A point regarding input devices and comfort is that many of the devices other than the mouse will require a learning period, so there may be an initial period in which workflow actually slows down before it speeds up with familiarity.

Once the telemedicine workstation and clinical environment have been optimized (see Chapter 3), the actual diagnostic process needs to be considered. It is important to know that a number of clinical specialties have telemedicine practice guidelines in place, and whenever possible these should be incorporated into any practice and followed whenever feasible and appropriate. In addition to technical requirements, these guidelines often provide protocols for acquiring proper diagnostic images (e.g., in teledermatology, which body parts should be imaged for particular diagnostic conditions); explaining procedures to patients and getting informed consent; protocols for what information to include in the patient referral history as well as in the diagnostic report; and cultural and diagnostic issues that might arise with special patient populations (e.g., pediatric, geriatric, mentally disabled). A systematic review of the literature also helps reveal what applications work better than others and what types of diagnostic protocols transfer readily to telemedicine or which ones require modification.

There are as many telemedicine consult protocols as there are programs, but there are some common features to all of them that contribute to successful consultations that do not unduly impose upon the normal workflow. Again, it can be very useful to contact other diagnostic telemedicine programs to find out what their protocols are and perhaps adapt them to your own unique situation. As noted previously, it is also important to evaluate and select peripheral devices that provide the best diagnostic quality information for the application being developed. For example, a high-end electronic stethoscope is probably required for telecardiology applications, but a middle-range one may be appropriate and sufficient for more general applications.

Nearly every step in the telemedicine diagnostic process involves human interaction, and thus human factors issues come into play at nearly every juncture and should be considered to ensure that the diagnostic process is as accurate as possible and the workflow as efficient as possible. Some of the key questions to consider from a personnel perspective when setting up a diagnostic telemedicine environment include the following: Who decides to refer a case to telemedicine? What is the procedure for referring a case? What is the procedure for consulting on a case? What kind of information does the teleconsultant require to render a diagnostic or treatment decision? Who organizes the case information, does the scheduling, manages the network connections, and facilitates the session? Some of these are more applicable to real-time sessions (scheduling), but in general apply to both store-and-forward and real-time situations.

Many programs have dedicated engineering and information technology teams to take care of the technical steps in a diagnostic telemedicine encounter and to troubleshoot problems that might arise. For many of the other steps (e.g., setting up consult sessions, collecting and processing patient record data), a dedicated site coordinator is often the point person. The role of the site coordinator often depends on the size of the program. Smaller programs with low volume may only need someone part time, whereas larger volume programs may require at least one full-time person. The qualifications of the site coordinator vary, but in general it is useful to have someone with at least some medical training or experience so they understand the language and culture of medicine. Technical skills are required as well because this person will likely be the one compiling the case, possibly acquiring the digital images, creating a case file on the computer, transmitting the case to the teleconsultant, and receiving the report back via the same computer. As this person will also likely be interacting with patients on a regular basis, he or she will need to have adequate interpersonal skills. With special patient populations such as older adults, it is even more important that the site coordinator have the necessary interpersonal skills to deal with the special considerations of these patients.

Most telemedicine consultations require paperwork to be filled out (either hardcopy or softcopy), and it is important to keep these forms as simple and straightforward as possible. With older patients it may often be easier to use hardcopy forms if the patient is not very familiar with using computers or other electronic input devices. Many forms can readily be adapted from existing forms used in traditional practice. In general, these forms fulfill medical, legal, and sometimes research requirements and must all be in place before a diagnostic teleconsult can take place. At a minimum, three forms are typically required. The first is informed consent, and this often includes information about the telemedicine encounter procedure, HIPAA, and other related security and privacy concerns. The second form typically collects basic patient information, including demographics and insurance information. The third form is a patient history form and generally requests details about the current problem, extent, duration, treatments tried, and so on.

Although a generic form suffices for many teleconsults, there are some specialties that have specific forms or questions related to that specialty (e.g., a teledermatology form may include a picture of the human body on which the patient can indicate where the skin problem is). These forms are generally filled out by the patient and collected, stored, and transmitted to the teleconsultant by the site coordinator or referring health care provider. In addition, pertinent adjunct information can be sent (and should be as often as possible). This includes relevant labs, progress notes, imaging reports, digital images, other consultation reports, hospital discharge summaries, and so on. The more information the teleconsultant has about the patient the better. This is especially true for store-and-forward consultations in which the teleconsultant does not have direct access to patients to probe them for more detailed information. Even for real-time teleconsultations, having as much information as possible in advance of the encounter is desirable because it prepares the consultant better and saves valuable time during the consult.

For store-and-forward teleconsultations the process is a little easier than for real-time sessions in the sense that it is not necessary to coordinate the schedules of the referring clinician, the consulting clinician, and the patient. Once the patient completes the paperwork, the onsite coordinator or health care provider explains the teleconsult procedure and the fact that the patient's information is going to be transmitted electronically to a specialist. The health care provider collects whatever other information is needed (e.g., for teledermatology, acquires the digital photographs using standard clinical practice guidelines) from the patient and then the patient is generally free to go home and wait for the results. The coordinator then finishes compiling the case, transmits it to the teleconsultant, and waits for the report to be returned (often using a specific form as well). The local health care provider then contacts the patient with the results and recommendations.

For real-time consultations, it is recommended that first-time patients arrive early, not only to fill out the required paperwork, but to meet the site coordinator or whoever will be conducting the session locally. This helps put patients at ease and gives them an opportunity to ask questions. It is also useful to take patients to the telemedicine room and familiarize them with the equipment and the format of the teleconsultation. For example, they will need to know where the camera is, where they should look, where the microphone is, etc. If peripheral devices are going to be used (e.g., electronic stethoscope, otoscope, handheld exam camera), it is useful to familiarize the patient with these as well. During this orientation the coordinator needs to be sensitive to generational and cultural issues. Older patients are likely to be less familiar with telecommunications technologies so may require more explanation and encouragement than younger patients who likely interact with electronic media on a daily basis. In terms of culture, for example, there are many cultures that prefer to utilize local health care providers such as shamans or medicine men instead of mainstream health care providers, so the site coordinator or telemedicine program should accommodate and embrace these customs as much as possible. In the Arizona Telemedicine Program, for example, each Native American telemedicine clinic that was established held an opening ceremony in which the local medicine man blessed the equipment and participants.

Basic videoconferencing etiquette should be reviewed with the patient—and will include all involved if they have not done a teleconsult previously. For example, patients need to be made aware that if the teleconsultant starts to talk they have to wait until they have finished speaking to avoid lost crossover audio signals. The patients often need to be reassured that the video is private, secure, and confidential. This is often especially true with older patients, who may not understand the technology and its capabilities. The key is to make the patient as comfortable as possible before the teleconsult even begins.

Once the real-time teleconsult begins, it is useful to start out with basic introductions and the teleconsultant confirming that the patient is comfortable and has no additional questions before starting. The actual flow of the diagnostic session depends on the clinical specialty, the problem, and the style of the teleconsultant. If peripheral devices are used during the consult, both the local coordinator and the teleconsultant should explain as much as possible to the patient with respect to what is happening, what data are being collected and why, and what the patient can expect to happen. In most real-time sessions it is preferred that a health care provider be present at the local site with the patients to reassure them, answer any questions during or after the session, and be prepared to implement whatever recommendations the teleconsult provides. Although the real-time teleconsultant often generates a report after the session, it may take a day or more for the referring site to receive it.

In general, there are two keys to setting up and running successful diagnostic telemedicine consultations. The first is to establish in advance as much of the protocol as possible, with assignments clearly delineated and responsibilities described to all involved. This will help with the altered workflow in general required to do telemedicine, but will also help with standardizing procedures as much as possible so that they soon become routine.

The second key is training—and more training. Before starting to conduct either store-and-forward or real-time teleconsultations, it is wise to obtain as much general training as possible and as much specific hands-on experience as well. All participants need to understand how the equipment works, what to expect in terms of performance, and what the limitations of the technology are. They also need to understand what the various requirements are for their role in the telemedicine encounter and what skill sets they need to have. The hands-on aspect is crucial, especially when technology is involved. Nearly everyone knows how to point and shoot with a digital camera, but a certain amount of skill is required to obtain useful diagnostic pictures of a skin lesion. Practice acquiring digital images and having them evaluated by the teleconsultant prior to any actual consultations is highly recommended. Mock real-time sessions are also quite useful, especially in specialties that require significant interaction with the patient, such as rheumatology and neurology, where gait or other motion tracking activities and tests (e.g., neck rotation) are involved. The more practice the participants have, the more likely the diagnostic teleconsultation will run smoothly and successfully.

6.3 Issues in Health Status Monitoring

In this section a brief tutorial is provided on the problem of detection of a critical health event. The move toward deploying health care devices in the home, under the control of health care users, raises many issues concerning how reliably such systems will perform.

6.3.1 Reliable Detection

The main goal of health status monitoring is to provide timely information about health status. The assumption is that health care costs can be minimized and quality of life maximized when adverse health conditions are identified and treated as early as possible. (Those assumptions are currently unresolved for some types of screening, such as for breast and prostate cancers.) In traditional health care, one waits for an individual to seek out help from a health care professional (or for a bystander to seek out help when the individual is unable to act). With remote monitoring, it is possible to identify changes that might not be recognized or reported by the monitored individual. No monitoring system is perfect, whether one considers the equipment or the human components. A series of trade-offs are usually made between sending too little or too much information.

Take the example of trying to detect falls via worn or carried equipment containing accelerometers that monitor acceleration and deceleration patterns over time. An algorithm is used to decide if a movement pattern indicates a fall. The problem is that there are patterns that are not falls but that resemble falls (e.g., sitting down quickly, flopping onto a bed, exercise activities). Any fall detection system therefore needs to define a threshold for sending an alert. The device could be programmed to be highly sensitive, but as a result might generate too many false alarm events, or it could be programmed to be less sensitive but might miss a real fall.

The problem is illustrated in Figure 6.2, which shows the two potentially overlapping frequency distributions, nonfall events (dotted line) and fall events (solid line). The *X*-axis represents the degree to which the event resembles a true fall, seen as increasing impact strength from left to right. (The *Y*-axis represents the frequency of occurrence, from low to high.)

As long as the two distributions, nonfall events and fall events, have some overlap, no matter where the criterion is set there can never be 100% reliability in fall detection (always reporting true falls and never reporting nonfalls). Imagine setting a very liberal criterion point (move the perpendicular criterion line to the left). Now the system will almost always report most fall events, but at the cost of reporting many nonfall events as falls. Imagine trying to reduce the number of instances that nonfalls are called falls by moving the criterion line to the right (more conservative criterion). Now few nonfall events will be reported as falls, but at the cost of missing many real fall events.

A diagram of the potential consequences that result from the situation shown in Figure 6.2 is evident in the 2 × 2 matrix shown in Table 6.1. The cells of the table represent frequencies of occurrence of joint events (fall and no fall crossed with whether a report was sent or not sent). Imagine that the system has been operating for a reasonable length of time and that there is independent confirmation of a fall event (perhaps by the monitored person or another observer).

Table 6.1 Matrix of Possible Events and Reports for Those Events

	Fall	No Fall
Report Sent	A: Correct Detection	B: False Alarm
No Report	C: Miss	D: Correct Rejection

It is possible to define how accurate the system is at fall detection by comparing various ratios (probabilities), such as sensitivity (correctly identifying true falls), specificity (correctly identifying true non-falls), positive predictive value (being accurate when a fall event is signaled), and negative predictive value (being accurate when a non-fall is not signaled). These ratios are defined as follows:

Sensitivity = a/(a+c)
Specificity = d/(b+d)
Positive Predictive Value = a/(a+b)
Negative Predictive Value = d/(c+d)

It is also possible to use prior information about the prevalence of falls in the population to estimate the likelihood that a fall occurred when a signal is sent. That is, one might have some baseline information about fall risk that can be factored into the event's interpretation (e.g., when a report is sent). Some medications (e.g., antipsychotics) are known to increase fall risk, so one might want to condition conclusions based on knowledge of such prior odds. Although they are beyond the scope of this primer, Bayesian statistics take prior probabilities into account for classifying an observed event. In practical terms, one would try to implement individual-based adjustment of the algorithm (basically, moving the criterion for reporting to the left or to the right).

6.3.2 The Problem of False Alarms

It may seem reasonable to select a very liberal criterion (perpendicular line in Figure 6.2 moved to the far left); that is, to report almost any potential fall event as a fall. If the system is not sensitive enough and misses falls, then it is not a very useful system. However, setting such a liberal criterion might lead to a very high rate of false alarms and a low positive predictive value for a signal being sent. Consistent with the fable of the boy who cried wolf, people might start ignoring reported events when their positive predictive value is very low. It also might prove quite costly to respond to a false alarm (e.g., send someone to the home to investigate).

To give one example, a 1994 study of a hospital pediatric intensive care unit (ICU) over a period of one week showed that fewer than 6% of alarms (of 2,176 observed) were clinically important, with a false alarm rate of 68% and an induced rate (false alarm through accidental triggering) of 26%. The positive predictive value of an alarm varied between 3% and 16% for the various devices being used (pulse oximeter, end-tidal PCO2, ventilator, EKG). Imagine a health care worker assigned to that ICU and that an alarm occurs. How quickly would the person respond when more than 9 times out of 10 it turned out to be a false alarm? That is, there is a nontrivial cost to signaling the presence of critical events when they are false alarms, both in terms of fatiguing health care workers and having them respond slowly to, or even ignore, true critical events.

The best way to minimize false alarms is to ensure that the algorithms used for detection have both high specificity and sensitivity. In terms of Figure 6.2, a more sensitive detection device effectively pushes the two curves farther apart so that they have little (or ideally no) overlap. This is easier said than done. One way to accommodate individual differences for a given instrument's fixed sensitivity and specificity is to tune parameters based on the older adult's risk profile. So, for instance, for fall detection, if the person is relatively inactive, one might set a more liberal criterion for registering an impact event as a fall because any severe impact is unlikely to be the result of normal, slow movement by the senior (hence, move the criterion line in Figure 6.2 to the left before reporting a fall). For someone who is a very active senior, adopt a more conservative criterion (move the criterion line for reporting to the right) to ensure that visits to the health club don't trigger a batch of false alarms. Of course, these issues need to be discussed with the individual being monitored (and their caregivers) to ensure that appropriate decisions are made and that the costs and benefits are fully discussed and understood.

6.4 *Suggested Readings*

Burroughs, C.M. & Wood, F.B. (2000). *Measuring the Difference: Guide to Planning and Evaluating Health Information Outreach.* Bethesda, MD: National Library of Medicine.

Grady, B., Myers, K., & Nelson, E. (2009). American Telemedicine Association's practice guidelines for videoconferencing-based telemental health. Retrieved from http://www.americantelemed.org/files/public/standards/Practice-GuidelinesforVideoconferencing-Based%20TelementalHealth.pdf.

Krupinski, E.A., Burdick, A., Pak, H., et al. (2007). American Telemedicine Association's practice guidelines for teledermatology. *Telemedicine & eHealth,* 14, 289–302.

Krupinski, E.A., Williams, M.B., Andriole, K., et al. (2007). Digital radiography image quality: Image processing and display. *Journal of the American College of Radiology,* 4, 389–400.

Lewis, J.R. (2006). Usability testing. In Handbook of Human Factors and Ergonomics, 3rd ed. G. Salvendy, ed., pp. 1275–1316. New York: John Wiley & Sons.

Olney, C.A. & Barnes, S. (2006a). *Getting Started with Community-Based Outreach.* Seattle, WA: National Library of Medicine.

Olney, C.A. & Barnes, S. (2006b). *Including Evaluation in Outreach Project Planning.* Seattle, WA: National Library of Medicine.

Olney, C.A. & Barnes, S. (2006c). *Collecting and Analyzing Evaluation Data.* Seattle, WA: National Library of Medicine.

Stronge, A.J., Nichols, T.A., Rogers, W.A., & Fisk, A.D. (2008). Systematic human factors evaluation of a teledermatology system within the U.S. military. *Telemedicine and e-Health,* 14, 25–34.

Williams, M.B., Krupinski, E.A., Strauss, K.J., et al. (2007). Digital radiography image quality: Image acquisition. *Journal of the American College of Radiology,* 4, 371–388.

chapter 7

Tutorial on Conducting Focus Groups

In this chapter focus group methodology is introduced and guidelines are presented for running a successful focus group study.

7.1 What Are Focus Groups?

It has been stressed throughout this text that it is important to understand and appreciate from a variety of perspectives the person(s) who will be utilizing the technologies and systems that make telehealth what it is. Not only is it important to understand and characterize physical and cognitive limitations or challenges, but it is important to understand user attitudes and expectations. Without actually involving people, there is no "human" in human factors or usability analyses. The question, of course, is how do we actually get those data?

One key method for assessing opinions and attitudes about a particular topic or device (e.g., wearable motion sensors to detect falls) or getting feedback about a particular device or application is the focus group. Focus groups are very useful in human factors research as they allow, for example, the designers of a device to preview it to the intended audience, let them interact with it, and get immediate feedback for future optimization and revision. For example, a focus group to get feedback on a wearable telemetric ECG device for older patients with irregular heartbeats may specifically want to get feedback about the weight of the system and the texture/comfort of the material used in the device, since skin sensitivity and allergies can change with age and the material used for something to be used by older patients may need to be different than for younger patients.

Focus groups fall under the general rubric of qualitative research and are valuable sources of information. Typically a group of interest is recruited, presented with some sort of scenario, product, or other topic of interest, and then encouraged to interactively and freely discuss their opinions with the other group members. Usually it is necessary to convene more than one group on a particular topic to get the full spectrum of feedback. About 3–4 usually suffices. Once the information starts to get redundant from one session to the next, it is usually time to stop.

A facilitator is usually present to help present the problem, lay down the ground rules for interaction, and keep the group focused and on track, but otherwise does not try to actively guide or direct the content of the conversation in any particular direction. Focus sessions are typically recorded in some fashion so the content can be reviewed, compiled, and organized after the session is closed.

7.2 Getting Started

Before convening a focus group, it is crucial to go through some key preparatory steps to help ensure the success of the session. The first step is to clearly define the purpose of the focus group and the key objectives. It is important to keep these as concise and clearly defined as possible and guide the rest of the planning and execution of the session around these core objectives. Without a clear purpose and statement of goals, the session is likely to be unfocused and meandering, and will yield little in terms of meaningful or useful data.

Defining the goals should be done by all of the key stakeholders in the process. For example, if the focus group is going to gather opinions and feedback about a wearable telemetric ECG sensor for older patients with irregular heartbeats, it would be useful to include perhaps the system designers, engineers, a cardiologist, a nurse, and a financial person in the objectives development phase in order to cover the full spectrum of variables that might affect the future development, marketing, and use of the device.

Once the objectives are defined, it should be clear who the intended audience should be, and thus identification of the focus group participants should readily evolve. Again, it is important to be as precise as possible in defining the focus group participants. Although estimating statistical power is important in quantitative research, it is much harder in qualitative research. It is, however, important to decide how many participants you need. There are no set rules for this, but it is important to get a sufficient number of participants to get a broad spectrum of opinions, but the group should not be so big as to be unwieldy and not conducive for everyone to interact. A group of about 6–12 participants is usually a good size. Fewer than 6 tends to limit conversation as well as group diversity, while more than 12 gets too unwieldy, especially in terms of letting everyone get a chance to speak. If more people are required for some reason, it would be useful to consider multiple smaller groups rather than one very large group. Although group diversity is important, it is also important to be somewhat homogeneous in terms of general characteristics as they pertain to the goals. For example, if you are getting feedback about a telemetric wearable ECG device for older patients, it is important to limit the participants to those likely to use it—older patients with irregular heartbeats as opposed to general cardiology patients of various ages and conditions. (When relevant candidates are difficult to obtain and each individual opinion counts, a hybrid procedure could be considered. It would entail having an individual interview first, followed by group discussion, though this can be quite costly in time.) It is generally a good idea to over-invite and expect a 10%–20% no-show rate, though seniors do tend to be more reliable than younger adults.

Once the characteristics of the participants are defined, it is necessary to determine how they will be recruited. This may require the cooperation of someone outside your organization, such as a physician at a heart clinic, the administrator at a retirement community, or the nurse at a facilitated living complex. If incentives are going to be offered for participation, they should be defined in advance and noted in the recruitment materials. The recruitment materials should be clear and designed appropriately for the targeted participant group in terms of language, reading level, and legibility (e.g., font size and contrast). Many institutions (not just academic) are likely to require Internal Review Board (IRB) Human Subjects review and approval of the project, so it is important to take care of this in advance of any active recruitment. At the very least, a consent form should be created and filled out by all participants prior to the session. The recruitment materials should also include the time commitment expected on the part of the participants. With older participants this is especially important as they may be relying on set modes and schedules of transportation rather than using an independent means of getting around.

It is important to also consider the focus group location, and this may be particularly relevant with older participants. Any focus group location needs to be large enough to accommodate the group without being so big that they feel like they are in a cave. Familiar, easily accessible locations are preferred. The participants need to feel comfortable, so choosing the right lighting, seating, acoustics, and general ambiance is important. The room acoustics and lighting are important so as to accommodate deficits in vision and hearing. With older participants it is also necessary to consider how they will get there, since many of them may not drive or may require assistance with wheelchairs, walkers, and the like. Parking should be close and readily available. If there are parking fees, ways to reimburse or cover them for participants should be considered, especially for those living on fixed incomes. If possible, it is useful with older participants to choose a meeting location where many may already meet, such as a community center.

Before the focus group meets, it is necessary to create a series of questions to guide the interaction. For a session lasting 1–2 hours there will only be enough time to really address about 4–7 questions, and this takes into account the time used initially to welcome the group, review the purpose, define the goals, and demonstrate any aspects of the topic or device the session is about. The best questions are open-ended and move from general to specific. The questions should not be leading questions so as not to bias the conversation. For example, instead of asking participants what they like about the wearable ECG sensor concept, the question could be more along the lines of, "if you were designing a wearable ECG, what properties would be important for you?" Usually the question generation process will yield more questions than can be addressed in an hour or two, so it is useful to go back to the key objectives and review how well the questions match or address those objectives. If they do not match, then they should be eliminated. Every session will have a different pace, so it is always better to have a few more questions available than too few. If they are prioritized in advance, then it is likely that the key ones will be addressed. The questions should be concise, to the point, unambiguously worded, open-ended, nonthreatening or nonembarrassing, and not amenable to short responses (e.g., yes/no). In some cases it may also be desirable to create a short (half-page) set of demographic questions for participants to fill in.

It is recommended that a script be developed prior to the session. The script should include a rough time line in addition to the order in which events are going to take place. It is not always necessary to write out a detailed scripting of the introduction, etc., but key ideas and wording of the questions should be established in advance. It is important to include a wrap-up section as well that not only thanks the participants for coming, but reiterates what the next steps are in the process so they understand what happens next and whether they can receive feedback or further information about the results of the session.

Identifying a facilitator is important. There are professional facilitators that can be hired to run the sessions, but they are not always required if there is someone in your group who is familiar with the process and comfortable guiding the group, knows how to deal with both outspoken and shy participants, and knows how to keep the discussion on track. The facilitator need not be intimately involved with the project, but needs to be quite familiar with it. One reason is that one of the facilitator's jobs is to not only put the question out for discussion, but to regularly summarize and reflect back to the group the nature of the discussion to help with clarity and to avoid redundancy. An assistant facilitator should be present at the session as well to help with recording, passing out materials, and to help with summarizing. With an older group, this person could also help with assisting participants get seated, find/get to the restrooms, etc.

7.3 Conducting the Session

The session location needs to be set up prior to the participants arriving. The chairs should be arranged (a circle or u-shaped is usually best);

refreshments set out; lighting set; recording devices put in place and ready to go (stereo recording is very helpful for transcription purposes); name tags ready and laid out; and flip charts, white boards, and other presentation materials put in place. Once the participants arrive, the facilitator should welcome everyone, review the goals, the procedure, and the rules for engagement. They should also note that the session will be recorded and how, possibly pointing out the equipment. It is often useful to have the participants introduce themselves and possibly give a short statement about themselves and their interest in attending. It should also be stressed before the session begins that the session and all subsequent handling of the information collected are confidential, and how confidentiality will be maintained should be explained. Participants should also be reminded that their presence is voluntary and they can choose to participate or not, stay or leave without any negative repercussions.

Once the session starts, it is important to keep the tone positive, make sure everyone gets the opportunity to speak, get full answers (if necessary, the facilitator can draw out more information), keep track of time, and stay on track. With older participants it may be necessary to incorporate more break periods than one would with a younger group, especially if the session is closer to 2 hours than 1 hour in length.

The session itself has three key phases that should be guided by the script. Phase I is the opening where welcomes are made, purpose and goals reviewed, introductions made, and procedures defined. Phase II is the question section, using the questions developed prior to the meeting. Phase III is the closing, where thanks are given to the group and means for future input and how the data will be used are explained.

7.4 After the Session

A good focus group, one that generates useful information, is more than just a casual gathering of people having a general discussion about a topic. A good focus group takes planning and attention to details before, during, and after the meeting. The process after the meeting, although less time constrained in some respects, is perhaps the most intense. The goal of the postmeeting phase is to consolidate, organize, and analyze the data collected. There is no single method to accomplish this, but the general process is quite similar no matter what final analysis method is chosen.

Immediately following the session, the facilitator and any other organizers should write down or record any immediate impressions or comments they may have. The first formal step is almost always transcription of the recorded session, although it is important to view/listen to the recordings as well as to read the transcription, as much information can be derived from facial expressions, gestures, and tones of voices. For human factors research this is particularly important, as watching the participants interact with a device may be more useful than listening to their comments. For example, aging patients may be so used to simply moving a device further away or closer to be able to clearly see the buttons or text that they may not mention that the interface was visually less than optimal. But if the designer sees a number of participants doing this, it is clear that adjustments in the user interface should be made.

Once the transcription is ready, any notes taken during the focus group session should be integrated into the document. To help organize the material, it is generally useful to attribute each entry to a given participant using a coding system. The code helps transfer individual comments to a data spreadsheet if the process is to be automated. Coding of the data also helps maintain the confidentiality of the participants.

Once the transcript data are coded and organized, the analysis process can begin. This phase should really be conducted by at least two people experienced in qualitative analysis techniques. Using one person can lead to bias, which should of course be avoided. If only two key people are available for the analysis phase, a third person could be useful for resolution of disagreements between the two primary analyzers.

Again, there are various techniques to use, but core to all of them is an attempt to find common categories or themes in the responses given to the questions posed during the session. Once the categories are agreed upon, the comments can be coded according to category and then sorted as a function of frequency of responses in a given category for each question. Once this is accomplished, it is useful to write a short summary paragraph for each category, including any prototypical or powerful quotes from the session. These summaries then form the basis for any reports or papers to be generated from the focus group sessions.

The final step is to bring the key stakeholders back together to go over the report and then develop action items and future steps based on the outcomes. Although the written report is useful, it quite often just gets filed without being read—defeating the purpose of the entire exercise.

7.5 Suggested Reading

Farley Templeton, J. (1994). *The Focus Group: A Strategic Guide to Organizing, Conducting and Analyzing the Focus Group Interview*. New York: McGraw-Hill.

Krueger, R.A. & Casey, M.A. (2000). *Focus Groups: A Practical Guide for Applied Research*. Thousand Oaks, Calif.: Sage.

Mitzner, T.L., Boron, J.B., Fausset, C.B., Adams, A., Charness, N., Czaja, S.J., Dijkstra, K., Fisk, A., Rogers, W.A., & Sharit, J. (2010). Older adults talk technology: Their usage and attitudes. *Computers in Human Behavior*, 26, 1710–21.

chapter 8

The Future, Resources, and Conclusions

We can expect continual improvements in telehealth technology in the coming decades in hardware and software interfaces and probably in instructional support. This chapter attempts to sketch out trends over the coming decade or two and highlight associations that provide useful information to practitioners.

8.1 Keeping the Promise of Human Factors Engineering: Promoting Efficiency, Safety, and Comfort

A careful consideration of the abilities of older adults both as providers and users of telehealth technology should lead to designing telehealth systems and environments that are efficient, safe, and enjoyable to use. Older providers may be able to practice their craft longer (e.g., through telesurgery) and older health care users may be able to maintain better health. Assessing efficiency, particularly cost effectiveness relative to traditional methods of providing care, remains an important area for research. Improving safety, in light of the Institute of Medicine report on error, continues to be a critical challenge, and will become even more salient as more health care services relocate into the less-standardized home environment.

8.2 The Future: Smart Homes, Remote Monitoring, and Treatment

The future of telehealth development lies in two broad areas: monitoring and treatment. The former will include better remote monitoring, and the latter will include education, treatment, and rehabilitation. Better monitoring and treatment will entail interacting with people where they live, rather than having them come into offices, clinics, and hospitals, except as a last resort or for certain complex tests and procedures.

The infrastructure to support telehealth continues to improve by leaps and bounds, as seen in the widespread deployment of high capacity transmission channels, ranging from wired broadband to an increasing proportion of homes (about 60% of homes in the United States in 2010) to higher capacity wireless networks serving the miniaturized computers called smartphones and tablets. It is no longer a spectacular feat to send a medical image in real time from a machine to a remote site or to share a stored image with remote consultants. The cost of processing and transmitting health care data continues to drop sharply.

It seems highly likely that health care technology, as it standardizes, will eventually be incorporated into homes, apartments, and other forms of congregate housing in the same way that plumbing, electrical wiring, wired telephone, and television cable systems are now deployed. Today there are many examples of smart homes that attempt to build in new health care functionality. One interesting concept being explored is the home as a "coach" for its inhabitants, encouraging occupants to pursue healthier lifestyles. Artificial intelligence systems, including intelligent robots, have a role to play in making this happen.

However, there is always a considerable lag between invention, commercialization, and adoption. The fax machine took about 150 years from invention to widespread dissemination. The wired telephone took about 50 years. The Internet enjoyed widespread adoption in about 20 years. So the pace of deployment and adoption is speeding up. However, the current stock of housing will be with us for many years to come. Thus retrofitting telehealth technology into existing structures will be a major focus for the 21st century. There are many challenges to meet in integrating telehealth technologies into older homes, apartments, and chronic care residences. One possibility being actively explored is to build a "telehealth station," a mini-clinic, into a dedicated room in a building, for instance in an apartment complex. People could visit this room to have vital signs monitored and perform other health checkup routines. Still, the ideal might be to have telehealth stations deployed in individual apartments and homes as costs for such equipment decline.

As sensors continue to improve, particularly in terms of their range of functions, sensitivity of detection, and size, they will increasingly be deployed in homes and, literally, on and in people to stream health data to health care providers. Many such systems have already been developed, particularly for monitoring vital functions such as pulse–oxygen, blood glucose, weight, and activity (e.g., detecting falls). A key concern will be automating such systems to a greater extent (so-called passive monitoring) such that users will not need to interact much with them, except for maintenance purposes, such as changing or recharging batteries. Of course, with automation comes the risk of overreliance on potentially fallible hardware and software. For person to person interaction, videoconferencing is becoming more widely available using inexpensive off-the-shelf computers equipped with cameras, and increasingly via smartphone systems (though the size of smartphone screens may be a barrier for older adults with vision problems, so intermediate devices such as tablet systems may be preferable). But too often such technology is designed without considering older adult capabilities, both for use and in terms of the training requirements. Although we can rely on markets to eventually weed out truly bad design, it would be far better to get the design right in the first place.

In summary, we are indeed entering a "brave new world" with respect to telehealth technology. Hopefully users, particularly older users, will have to be neither brave nor very physically or cognitively fit to be able to take advantage of its benefits. The goal of this volume has been to provide relevant pointers and guidelines to good design.

8.3 Associations Devoted to Human Factors and Telehealth

The International Ergonomics Association coordinates human factors efforts worldwide: http://www.iea.cc/. In the United States, the Human Factors and Ergonomics Society (HFES; www.hfes.org) is an excellent resource for human factors information, including a health care technical group (www.hfes.org/hctg) concerned with issues such as medical systems, patient safety, and rehabilitation.

The American Telemedicine Association (ATA) (www.americantelemed.org) is the premiere source of information on telemedicine. Although much of its material is restricted to members, some is available to the public. Joining the association provides full access to its white papers, guidelines, etc. There is also a special interest group in ATA on human factors.

Another organization with interests in this topic is the American Medical Informatics Association (AMIA; https://www.amia.org/). There are a number of working groups within AMIA that focus on topics relevant to human factors issues such as informatics, education, evaluation, ethical issues, and organizational issues. Relevant International Organisation for Standards (ISO) information for health care equipment can be found at http://www.iso.org/iso/iso_catalogue.htm, and for the United States, the Food and Drug Administration (FDA) requirements can be found at http://www.fda.gov/MedicalDevices/default.htm.

8.4 Conclusion

The world's population is aging, relatively quickly in developed countries and somewhat more slowly in developing ones. Increased age is associated with increased morbidity, due primarily to the onset of chronic disorders. Health care spending represents a large and growing percentage of national welfare expenditures, and chronic care accounts for a very high percentage of those health care expenditures. Telehealth technology is a promising tool for providing high quality and hopefully cost effective health care to an aging population, as long as the telehealth systems are easy to use by both aging practitioners and their aging health care clients.

To ensure that these systems are usable and useful, it is necessary to pay close attention to human factors. Our book supplies basic information about how aging affects human capabilities that are essential to successful interaction with such systems. We have also discussed the range of telemedicine applications that are in use and in development. We have provided tips about how best to install and use such systems. Because technology continually advances, we have focused on guidelines and principles that should apply not just to existing but also to future systems. We have also reviewed human factors techniques such as usability testing and focus group testing that are essential for ensuring that these systems can be deployed, used, and maintained successfully. We hope that this book will play a useful role in facilitating the provision of safer, more efficient, and more comforting health care to present and future aging populations.

8.5 Suggested Readings

Carayon, P. (2007). *Handbook of Human Factors and Ergonomics in Health Care and Patient Safety*. Hillsdale, N.J.: Lawrence Erlbaum Associates.

Weinger, M.B., Wiklund, M.E., & Gardner-Bonneau, D.J. (2010). *Handbook of Human Factors in Medical Device Design*. Boca Raton, FL: CRC Press.

Index

D

E

F

G

H